To Mama & Adam

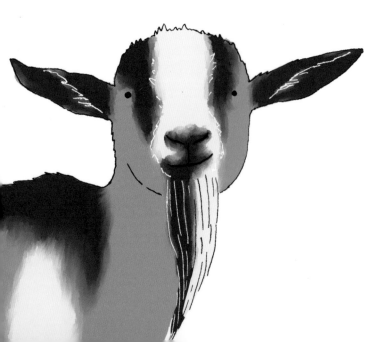

SARA BOTERO

THE ESSENTIAL
VEGAN
toolkit

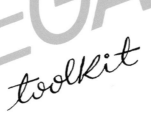

LIMINAL 11

This edition published in 2020 by Liminal 11

First published in 2019 by Liminal 11

Written and illustrated by Sara Botero

This edition published in 2020 by Liminal 11

Cover and book design by Sara Botero

Printed in Turkey

ISBN 978-1-912634-20-0

10 9 8 7 6 5 4 3 2 1

www.liminal11.com

DISCLAIMER: The information provided in this book is of a general nature and is
for information purposes only. We've made every effort to ensure accuracy, but this
information is not to be taken as advice regarding any health or medical conditions.
Please consult your physician before making any major changes to your diet.

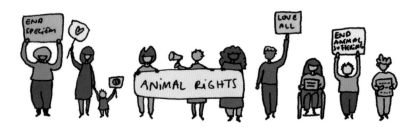

"Veganism is a way of living which seeks to exclude, as far as is possible and practicable, all forms of exploitation of, and cruelty to, animals for food, clothing or any other purpose."

THE VEGAN SOCIETY

WELCOME TO MY BOOK!

INTRODUCTION

We live in a world where vegan isn't the standard way of living, so this book aims to help you along the way. This book is for:

-Those looking to find out what veganism is about and reasons to go vegan.
-For those who are already on the road to becoming vegan.
-For those who are already vegan but like to have a book full of handy and easy-to-read information all in one place.

Whether you want to be an overnight vegan or you want to take it one step at a time, I hope this book helps you on your vegan journey.

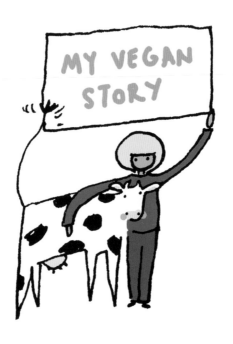

I studied environmental science at the University of Reading and in my final year I transitioned to veganism. Originally I was only planning on going vegetarian because I thought veganism was a bit extreme! However, my views were changed when I met my first ever vegan and she became my friend. I saw and ate the amazingly delicious, easy food she made and also had conversations about animal rights, such as how can you humanely kill an animal?

However, I still ate products with dairy in them as I didn't think I was contributing to animal cruelty. I quickly realised that this was another form of disassociation, so I quit dairy and ate a lot of Oreos instead.

Eggs were one of the final animal products to go. I soon learned how to make huevos rancheros with tofu and my mind was blown by how good they tasted. Now that I had a replacement for my Colombian dish cravings, no more eggs were broken! I soon quit eating honey after looking more into why it's bad for the bees and the environment.

I quickly spotted a pattern: when I wasn't letting go of something it was because I didn't know why I should. Some people can intrinsically understand that it's not theirs to take and some need a bit more information on the *why*. Hopefully this book will give you both the *why* and the *how* on veganism.

PART 1

Why Go Vegan

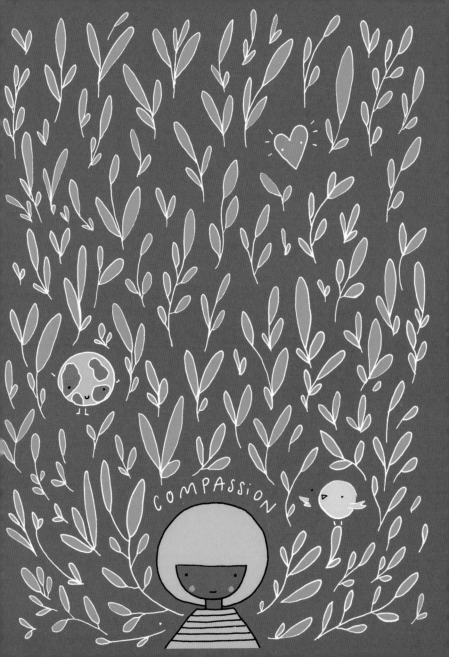

WHY GO VEGAN?

It is important to find a *why* to give you motivation like with anything in life. Different people have different reasons why they are vegan or want to go vegan. Sometimes it is just one reason and sometimes it is a multitude of reasons.

The following chapters are going to be broken up into three different *whys*: the animals, our planet and our health.

It's always useful to find out the different *whys* that exist for veganism. After having read them all, one might resonate with you more, but knowing them all will help you in your vegan journey.

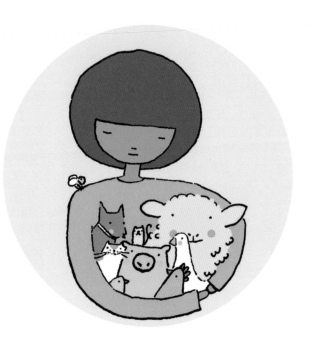

ANIMALS

One of the biggest reasons that people go vegan is because of the animals. Before I started to transition to veganism, I didn't know even a tiny portion of the atrocities that animals have to go through, simply because humans have found it convenient to exploit them for their own benefit.

We are compassionate beings and if we are given the chance to either cuddle a sheep or kill it, it's not really a difficult decision to choose to cuddle.

So why is it any different when we are given the choice of eating veggies instead of animals? The reason is that over time, with how animal products are marketed, we have been made to disassociate and are distanced from our true nature of wanting to cuddle instead of killing. So when we look at the burger on the menu we don't think about that animal suffering and dying so that it can be on our plate. Furthermore, in our society, eating animal products is very common, and when things are the "norm" we tend accept them without question. However, a lot of things in our society are normalised. Just because this is so doesn't mean they are right.

To stop the disassociation we must stop turning a blind eye for the sake of convenience. In the following chapter we will be covering the things that animals have to go through to end up being eaten or used by humans.

NATURAL LIFESPAN

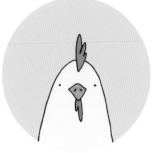

Chickens
For meat: 6 weeks
For laying eggs: 1-2 years
NATURAL LIFE SPAN:
Up to 8 years

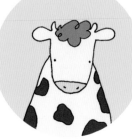

Cows
For 'beef': 18 months
For dairy: 4-5 years
Male dairy cows (used for veal): 1-24 weeks
NATURAL LIFE SPAN:
Up to 20 years

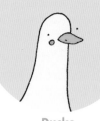

Ducks
For meat: 8-26 weeks
For laying eggs: 1-2 years
Male egg chicks: 1 day
NATURAL LIFE SPAN:
Up to 15 years

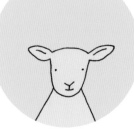

Lambs
For meat: 3-6 months
NATURAL LIFE SPAN:
Up to 12 years

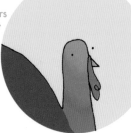

Turkeys
For meat: 8-26 weeks
NATURAL LIFE SPAN:
Up to 10 years

OF FARM ANIMALS

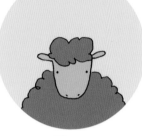

Sheep
For milk: 5 years
For breeding: 3 years
For wool: 7 years
NATURAL LIFE SPAN:
Up to 20 years

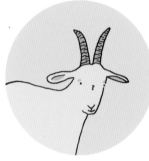

Goats
'Meat goat': 3-4 months
For dairy: 5 years
NATURAL LIFE SPAN:
Up to 18 years

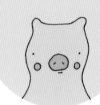

Pig
Slaughter age: 6 months
NATURAL LIFE SPAN:
Up to 15 years

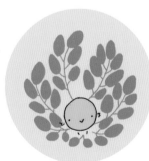

Male egg chicks
Slaughter age: 1 day
NATURAL LIFE SPAN:
Up to 8 years

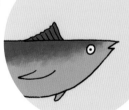

Fish
Farmed: less than a year
NATURAL LIFE SPAN:
Up to 15-30 years

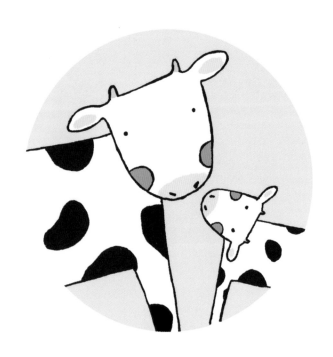

COWS

Cows are amazing creatures. They are caring, inquisitive, playful, clever and incredibly social beings. Cows communicate by touch, smell, vocalisations and body language. Cows are highly social so being isolated causes them psychological stress.

Dairy Cows

Cows are mammals just like us, so for them to lactate they need to either be pregnant or have been recently. For this to happen they need to be impregnated, and the farmer does this by inserting their arm into the cow's anus so as to relax the muscles of the vagina and then they are artificially inseminated. When the baby calf is born they are separated from their mother. If it's a male they get killed for veal; 112,000 dairy calves were killed in the UK in 2017. If they are female then they are destined for the same life of a dairy cow as their mother. In nature, mother and calf stay together for 9 to 12 months before being weaned; however in the dairy industry, separation often occurs within 3 days as to prevent mother and calf from bonding, the stronger the bond the more stress both mother and calf endure. Mother and baby experience terrible grief and can be heard calling for each other for long periods of time. As soon as three months, the cycle starts again for the mother cow, having to endure up to 4 to 5 times of giving birth and being separated from her baby.

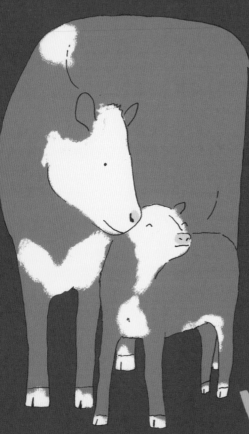

WE DIDN'T ASK TO BE BORN INTO A WORLD OF SUFFERING

In the 1800s a cow produced an average of 1000 litres of milk annually; the average now is 10,000. This is because cows have been bred by humans to produce unnatural amounts of milk, up to 10 times more. The weight of carrying that volume of milk is not only painful but also leads to infections such as mastitis. The current incident rate is 30+ cases per 100 cows. Mastitis causes the udders to swell or harden. This type of infection is so common that there are legal limits of how much pus is allowed in milk to be sold for human consumption. Dairy cows also quite commonly suffer from lameness due to the conditions that they are kept in and the prevalence of infections such as foot rot.

After four years their milk production declines. They are deemed unprofitable and are sent to the slaughterhouse, when they could have lived to be over 25 years old. Often they are so exhausted by the vicious cycle of being impregnated, giving birth, being separated, milked, impregnated and so on that their legs can't carry them any more and they fall to the ground. In the industry they are labelled as "downers" or "spent".

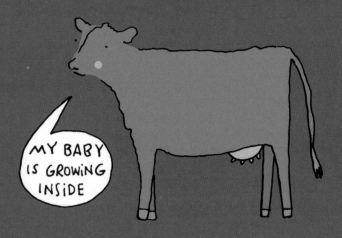

150,000 DAIRY COWS ARE
SLAUGHTERED WHILST PREGNANT
EACH YEAR IN THE UK

Cows farmed for meat

In their first week of being alive a baby cow will go through painful procedures such as de-horning & castration. De-horning is done so as to prevent the growth of horns. It is done either by using a hot iron or by applying a chemical. Both procedures are burning the bud, and the skin around it can also be burnt. Research has shown that all methods cause pain to the calves. De-horning also occurs in the dairy industry. In the UK there are three ways that a cow can be castrated; a rubber ring can used to cut off the circulation to the testicles, the spermatic cord can be crushed or they can be surgically removed. The first two options are legally allowed to be performed without any pain relief. Instead of the 25 or more years that they could live they are killed between 1 and 2 years old. Cows raised for both dairy and meat end up being transported to the slaughterhouse, where they are stunned with a bolt gun before being grabbed by their legs, lifted up and having their throats slit.

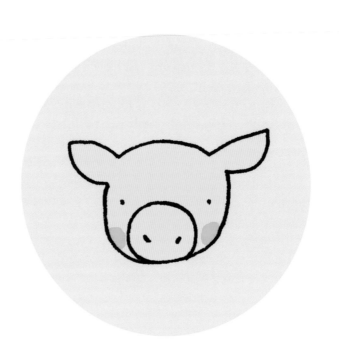

PIGS

Pigs are highly intelligent animals, more intelligent than dogs and three-year-old human babies. They are also very social and can express empathy. They can live up to 10-15 years, but factory-farmed pigs are sent to slaughter after just 4 to 6 months.

Pigs used for breeding are continuously impregnated. They are bred to have larger litters than what is natural. The mothers are pregnant for 115 days. In nature, weaning would be a gradual process of three to four months, but this doesn't happen when they are farmed and once separated they can be heard crying out for each other. In the UK gestation crates are no longer allowed; however, farrowing crates are still legal. This is where the mother is placed before giving birth. The mother's natural instinct is to make a nest but this behaviour is not possible in the small confinements of the metal bars. The farrowing crate doesn't even allow the mother to turn around to see to her piglets. The crate is also where she will nurse.

Between 3 and 4 weeks old piglets are taken from their mother. In some countries it's even earlier. Because the pigs are bred to have larger litters there isn't sufficient milk to go around, which creates competition for the best teat. To prevent injuries, piglets have their teeth clipped or ground down.

Even though tail docking is illegal in the EU, it still goes on. A UK report by the Agriculture & Horticulture Development Board (AHDB) found that 70% of pigs had their tails docked. This is done with heated pliers. If the piglet is less than a week old, anaesthetic or pain relief is not required. This is done to prevent tail biting; however, the tail biting happens because they are in stressful situations to begin with.

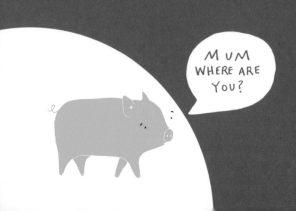

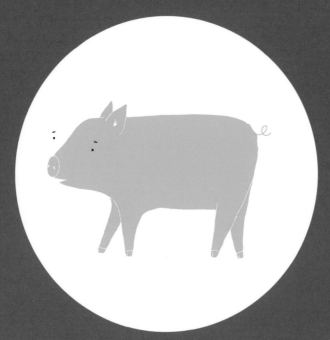

Male castration is not common in the UK because the pig is killed before they mature and develop "boar taint". However, it is still very common with roughly 90 million piglets being castrated every year in Europe (CIWF), and some of the meat gets imported into the UK. Many piglets get castrated without any anaesthetic or pain relief. This obviously causes them pain in the short term but also can lead to further health problems in the long term.

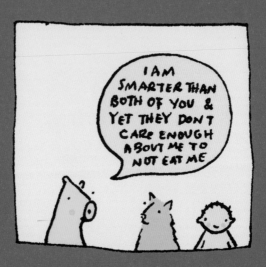

Pigs have to be transported to the slaughterhouse and often they have to travel long journeys without water to wherever the best price for them is on offer. Pigs only sweat through their snouts. The combination of this, lack of water and high temperatures means that they can suffer dehydration on their journey. Imagine being in the back of a lorry with other pigs, hearing unfamiliar sounds and traveling for hours on end, while stuck on a metal floor.

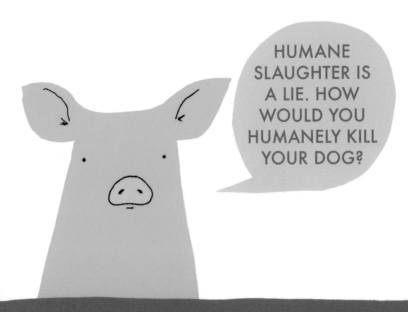

HUMANE SLAUGHTER IS A LIE. HOW WOULD YOU HUMANELY KILL YOUR DOG?

9 million pigs are slaughtered each year in the UK and 1 billion worldwide. It is not illegal for pigs to be killed in front of each other. They are stunned using electrocution through their brains or by being gassed. Both aren't guaranteed to be effective in stunning, with animal welfare investigation footage showing pigs gasping and trying to escape. They are then grabbed and hung from their back legs and their throats are slit.

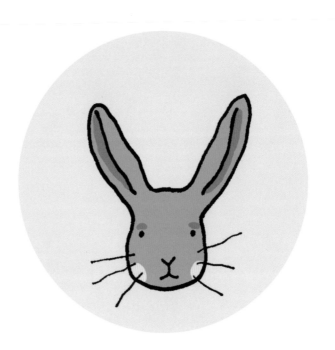

RABBITS

Rabbits communicate with each other with facial expressions and body language. Rabbits in the wild love to dig, can run up to 35 miles per hour and can jump over a metre high. They live in family groups of 3 to 12 plus their offspring. They live in a network of burrows underground, where there are different sections for different activities such as sleeping and eating. They are caring and spend a lot of time grooming each other. Sadly they are the second most farmed species in the EU and fourth in the world, with roughly 330 million rabbits slaughtered every year for their meat in the EU alone.

They don't get to perform their natural behaviours because most rabbits are intensively farmed. This means that they live their short lives squashed in with other rabbits with less space than an A4 piece of paper each. There is very little species-specific legislation to protect them. A rabbit can live between 10 to 15 years but when they are being raised for meat they are killed at 3 months old. Breeding rabbits (which are called does) are artificially inseminated while placed on their backs. This is incredibly traumatising to them because, as prey animals, being in such a vulnerable position goes against their natures. They produce litter after litter until the doe is classified as spent, then is killed at 18 months. Does and kits (young rabbits) are separated at 4 weeks old.

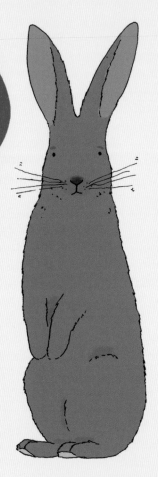

The cages that they are kept in have wire mesh flooring so that their excrement falls through; however, this mesh is very uncomfortable on their paws and can create lesions. Due to the unnatural way in which they are kept, disease and infections are common, which leads to a high mortality rate.

Some rabbits are killed on farms using methods such as: a blow to the head with a hammer, breaking their necks or being stunned first and then having their throats slit. Rabbits are naturally very frightful due to them being a prey animal, so being transported in loud conditions is very stressful for them. It is not a surprise that some die on the journey to the slaughterhouse. At the slaughterhouse they are hoisted onto a conveyor belt, electrically stunned and hung by their back legs to have their throats cut. Rabbits in the wild are either caught using a ferret and a net followed by having their necks broken or being shot, or they are shot from far away – the shot isn't always fatal so they die slowly.

Rabbits deserve to be free and not in a cage waiting to be killed. Did you know that when rabbits are happy, leap into the air and do a little twist?

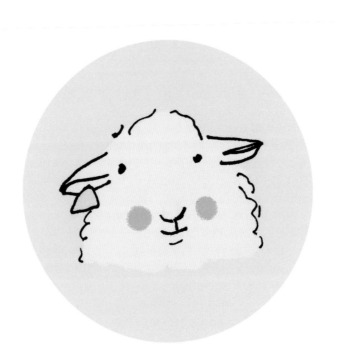

SHEEP

Sheep in the wild manage just fine by themselves. They shed their winter coat when spring comes just like dogs do, they graze for long hours wandering through the hills and they give birth to lambs in the spring time.

Things are very different for sheep that have been bred for humans to use as a commodity. They are selectively bred to maximise profit at the cost of their lives and freedom. They are bred to produce surplus wool, which leaves them susceptible to infections of fly-strike, where larva eat their flesh (read more in the section on wool, on page 70).

They are also bred to have multiple babies instead of the one that they would have normally. Ewes' natural behaviour is to give birth in spring time. Sadly, they are forced to give birth in winter so the farmer can sell the lambs for a higher price. However, this means that up to one fifth of young lambs don't survive. Sheep and their lambs form strong bonds and a mother can identify its baby's unique call. Imagine what it must feel like to be repeatedly grieving for babies that haven't even been weaned off, as well as then being separated from the ones that do survive!

If they do survive they have to endure ear-tagging and other mutilations such as castration and tail docking, both of which are incredibly traumatising and legally don't have to be performed with pain relief.

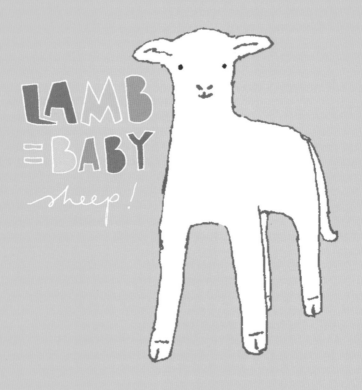

LAMB
=BABY
sheep!

Lambs' short lives come to an end at around 4 to 6 months by having to travel for long periods of time in noisy trucks, which due to their timid nature is very traumatising, instead of living for their natural lifespan of 12 years.

At the slaughterhouse there are two methods that are used to stun but not stop the heart so the sheep can be cut open and drained of their blood. One is a metal bolt that is shot into their brains and the other is an electrical rod to render them unconscious. However, undercover slaughterhouse footage shows that stunning is not always effective and they can regain consciousness whilst they are being bled to death.

Sheep are incredibly intelligent and caring. They can express emotions like we do, from joy to sadness. They are social beings and will nuzzle each other for comfort, jump for joy and hang their heads when sad. We wouldn't treat dogs like how we treat farm animals, so why should it be any different with any other sentient being?

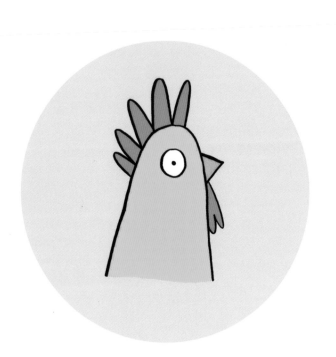

CHICKENS

The natural lifespan of a chicken can be up to 10 years, but when being raised for meat they are killed at 6 weeks old. Egg laying hens are killed when their production of eggs slows down at around 1-2 years old.

Chickens are intelligent animals that understand cause and effect and can solve complex problems. Mother hens start teaching different calls to their chicks whilst they are still in their eggs. They have roughly 30 different vocalisations to call their young, share information or send out an alarm call. When chicks are born, hens show affection to their babies and teach them what food they should eat and which ones to avoid.

Chickens like us experience REM sleep, which means that they dream when they're asleep.

Not only are chickens very smart and caring but, like us, they have a social hierarchy and can recognise up to 100 faces!

Hens in the wild will lay less than 20 eggs a year but this is not profitable so they have been bred to produce higher numbers of eggs. They are fed a high protein feed and left under lights to mimic daylight to force them to lay on average 500 eggs annually. This causes exhaustion and production decline, so they are killed at 1-2 years old because it's cheaper to bring in younger hens than to keep feeding the exhausted and unproductive hens.

In the UK alone more than 10bn eggs are produced each year! The RSPCA found that 48% of eggs produced in the UK, in 2017, came from battery cages. Whether the eggs are free range or organic, new egg-laying hen generations need to be bred to replace the tired out 2 year old hens. However, only the females are wanted for their reproductive organs, so the male chicks get ground up alive, gassed or suffocated at only one a day old.

Free range simply means that the chickens have access to outdoors for a certain number of hours per day. However, the barns are so cramped that they often don't even realise that there are doors to the outside. According to the RSPCA, free range eggs means that barns can legally contain up to 9 birds per square metre. This is equivalent to 14 adults living in a one-room flat.

Confining chickens in this way all their life means that they are incredibly distressed. Consequently, beak-cutting is a common mutilation practice to prevent cannibalism and feather pecking. This is done without anaesthetic. Debeaking is painful for the hens and they can have lifelong suffering because of it.

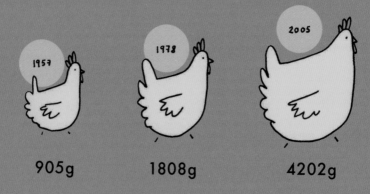

1957

905g

1978

1808g

2005

4202g

CHICKENS HAVE BEEN SELECTIVELY
BRED SO THAT THEY GROW AT AN
ACCELERATED RATE. SO MUCH SO
THAT THEIR YOUNG BONES CAN
BREAK DUE TO THE STRAIN OF
THEIR OWN WEIGHT.

Selective breeding for the purpose of maximising profits has meant that chickens grow so quickly that their legs cannot properly support their unnaturally large bodies. This leads to further health problems such as bone development abnormalities which are crippling and painful for the chickens and impair them from being able to move properly.

All chickens, whether they are bred for meat or eggs, end up at the slaughterhouse. They are grabbed by their legs and their world is turned upside-down, then they are shoved in small crates. It is legal for them to travel for long periods of time without any water or food.

They are shackled upside-down to a machine by their legs. A conveyor belt then transports them to a water tank, where they are electrocuted and lose consciousness, and then their throats are cut. The electrocution doesn't always work but regardless the conveyor belt continues.

Chickens are sweet, caring and intelligent beings who should be sunbathing with their friends and clucking at each other, not living a life of pain.

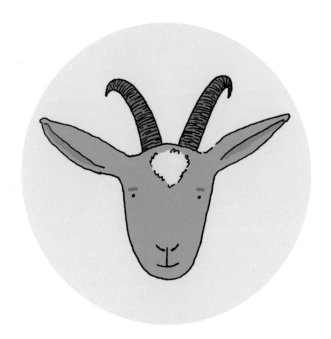

GOATS

Goats love to roam hills with other goats, as they are sociable beings who get depressed if left alone. Goats forage for long periods of time, up to 10 hours a day. Goats have a great sense of balance and can even climb trees! This is what they would normally do; however, when bred into the world for meat or dairy production, they don't get to experience this and instead are confined to a life in crowded feed-lots or – best case scenario – restricted pastures. When they would naturally cover a huge number of miles, it is no comparison.

Female goats fare the same cruel fate of dairy cows. Being continuously impregnated, having their babies taken away so that humans can drink their breast milk or turn it into cheese. At one week old the females have their horns burnt off; this is called de-budding. Male kids are 'surplus' to the dairy industry, like veal, so are slaughtered at 12 weeks old for meat.

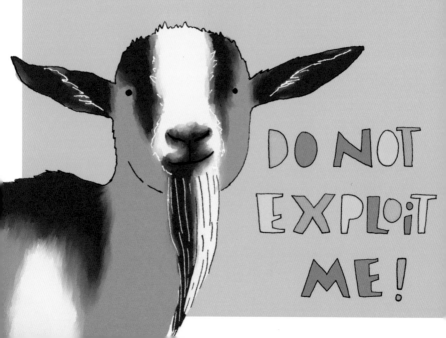

Goats raised for meat, whether they are female or male, undergo several mutilations at an early age. One of them is having their ears tagged and the other is de-budding, which is traumatic and incredibly painful. Male goats normally are castrated within a week of birth and it is performed with no pain relief. One of the methods is a tight rubber ring that is placed around the goat's testicles to cut off the blood supply.

Female goats are so nurturing that they will instinctively foster orphaned babies – not just baby goats but also calves and lambs. Animals are so full of love and compassion and they deserve that in return, instead of being harmed and eaten.

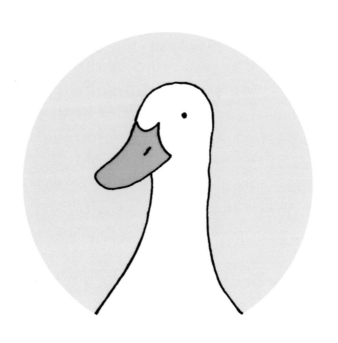

DUCKS

Ducks can live up to 20 years, but farmed ducks are killed at 7 weeks old. In the wild some ducks can fly up to 332 miles in a day!

We all know that ducks love water. In fact, when they are not kept in captivity, they spend 80% of their time in water. They do this because they are looking for food, and also because they use water to regulate their temperature and to prune themselves, which is crucial to them as this is how they keep themselves clean.

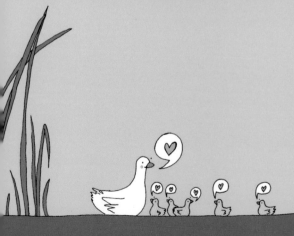

Ducks are bred for their meat, eggs and down. Most ducks bred for consumption are factory-farmed where they are crammed in with thousands of other ducks and have little to no access to water. Their feed and light is controlled to maximise weight gain.

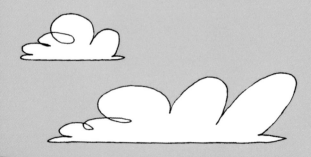

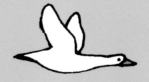

This rapid gain in weight can cause lameness, which means that the ducks can't support their own weight. Under these conditions diseases spread easily, killing not only ducks – mutated strains of their disease (avian flu) have also killed hundreds of humans. Ducks are also bred for their production of eggs and, like chickens, when their production declines they are sent to be killed.

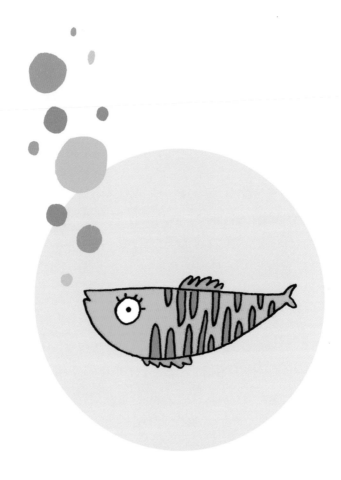

FISH

Fish feel pain.

Fish have a good memory.

Fish have been around since well before the dinosaurs. Fish are complex and intelligent animals, and some fish can even communicate with each other.

Some small fish, called cleaner fish, eat the dead skin off of bigger fish. It's good for the little fish because they get food and it's good for the big fish because they get cleaned. Scientists have observed that when the little fish accidentally nibbles too hard, the big fish experiences pain, and to reduce this the little fish gives them a back rub!

Fish feel as much as other non-human vertebrate. Just because fish aren't as cuddly as puppies, it doesn't mean that they should be treated without compassion.

Fish can feel pain, fish can remember, fish are complex and intelligent animals that have their own personalities.

Even though there is ever-increasing evidence that fish can feel pain we still treat them as if they can't. This means that there are no welfare laws enforced in the killing of fish at sea.

Nets catch thousands of fish at a time and the weight of the thousands of fish crush those at the bottom. This, and the change in pressure, causes their insides to be pushed out whilst they are still alive. If that doesn't kill them, they slowly suffocate to death on the boat's deck.

Nets catch more than just the fish they intend to catch. Each year it is estimated that over 20 million tonnes of marine life is caught and killed as bycatch. More than 300,000 of these individuals are whales, dolphins and porpoises.

Farming fish also has negative impacts on the fish and on other animals. They are reared intensively much like chickens or other farm animals are, with some sea cages holding up to 50,000 salmon.

This is the equivalent of a three-quarter metre salmon in a bathtub of water.

These cramped conditions cause stress to the fish, which leads to cannibalism and also creates a perfect environment for disease to spread, causing many fish to die. Diseases that originate from farmed fish who escape have wreaked havoc with wild fish populations.

Hundreds of seals have been reported as intentionally killed by fish farmers so as to protect their stock. Additionally, other marine animals as well as sea birds can get entangled in the nets and die or be injured. Conventional or organic fish are starved for 7 to 10 days before being killed. Most slaughter methods cause the fish to die slowly and painfully. These include: air asphyxiation, cutting them, CO_2 narcosis, ice bath, electrical stunning and knocking them dead.

Fish can feel pain. They show complex behaviour such as using tools and even giving massages after accidentally nibbling their host too hard as a way of stress relief. Fish don't belong on our plates. They belong in seas, rivers and lakes.

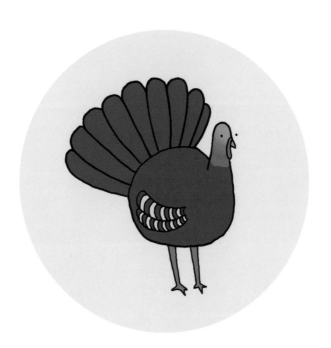

TURKEYS

Almost 630 million turkeys are produced for meat each year. They are selectively bred for fast growth and large breasts to increase profit with no regard for the pain of the turkeys. In the EU 90% are kept indoors in sheds that hold groups of up to 25,000 birds. As well as being bred to grow bigger and faster, they are also manipulated using light to make them eat as much as possible.

Due to the very fast and unnatural growth rate, turkeys are at high risk of lameness and other body defects. This causes them pain, difficulty in walking and they are no longer able to fly.

The waste from the birds contains ammonia, which impacts the quality of the air and can lead to respiratory and eye problems.

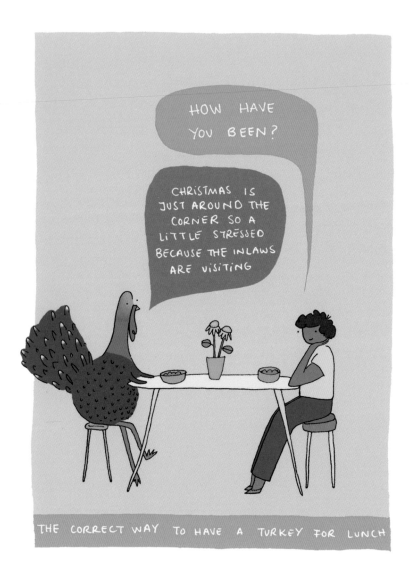

Keeping turkeys in overcrowded barns increases aggression and can lead to feather-pecking and cannibalism. For this reason some turkeys get their beaks trimmed when they are only days old, a procedure which is painful and traumatising. They are also kept in low light so as to diminish aggression; however, this can lead turkeys to develop eye abnormalities and blindness.

Turkeys are magnificent creatures who in nature will fly as fast 55mph and roost in trees. They are incredibly social and affectionate. They create friendships that last a long time, enjoy a good cuddle and when they are being petted they purr like cats do. They never get to live these experiences when their destination is somebody's plate.

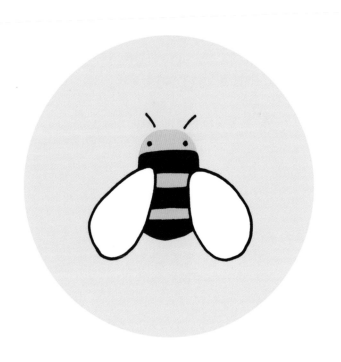

BEES

Honey bees produce honey for themselves. They have been doing this for millions of years. They have a highly complex society made up of the queen bee, a few thousand males and tens of thousands of female worker bees, some of whom are nurses and others foragers. The foragers do an intricate dance which communicates to the other bees the distance and location of good flowers and of any dangers.

They produce and store honey to last them through the winter. 1 teaspoon of honey is the life's work of 12 honey bees. In one day a bee can visit up to 5000 flowers. That is a heck of a lot of work!

Honey is bees' main source of nutrition. It is food nutritionally tailored for bees. This gets taken away from them and sold to humans. The honey is replaced with a sugar substitute to last them through the winter – in some extreme cases the hive is killed.

The queen bee is artificially inseminated and her wings are clipped to stop her from leaving. The rest of the hive won't leave as they are extremely loyal.

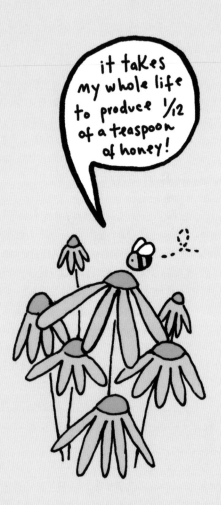

Not all bees produce honey. In fact there are about 20,000 different species of bees in the world and only 9 that produce honey. The most common honey bee is the European honeybee *Apis mellifera*. And did you know that bumble bees aren't honey bees?! Honey bees aren't endangered of going extinct but there are many other species which are. The majority of bees nest alone underground or in cavities.

The honey bee has been domesticated for our own benefit and it is not at risk. Quite the opposite: it poses risks to the population diversity of bees by creating competition for food and increasing diseases and parasites such as Varroa mite due to higher rates in commercial bees. Buying honey to conserve a bee species that is not at threat is flawed logic.

Instead here are some things that you can do: grow wild flowers that are native and drought resistant or/and let your lawn grow wild as "weeds" are great for bees. Don't use pesticides; if you can, buy organic. Say no to decking or concrete as solitary bees can't make a home there. Finally buy or DIY a bee hotel to provide more nesting sites. Simple changes can make a real difference.

ORGANIC / FREE RANGE

After reading the horrible facts about what animals have to go through to end up on our plates, you might be thinking 'well that's very well but I only buy organic/free range'. Organic and free range standards are supposed to be in place to improve the welfare of the animal and, with organic, for the human as well. For example, with organic meats, eggs and dairy, farmers are restricted in the amount of antibiotics and other pharmaceuticals that they are allowed to give to their livestock for the benefit of the consumer. However, this comes at the price of the chance that a suffering animal won't get the antibiotics that would make them feel better.

Furthermore, in organic farming these things still happen: male chicks in the egg industry still get destroyed, cows are forcibly impregnated over and over again and each time their baby gets taken away from them, chickens and cows in the egg and dairy industry will still end up being killed way before their natural lifespan.

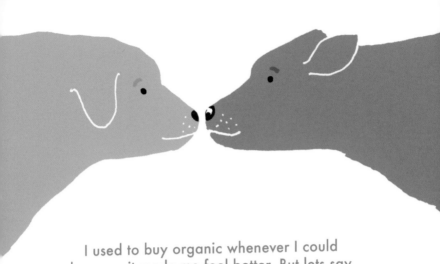

I used to buy organic whenever I could because it made me feel better. But lets say we swap a lamb for a puppy: the puppy gets some access to the outside and they aren't given growth hormones, but before their first birthday they are forced to travel long distances to the slaughterhouse where they will be electrocuted and their throats slit. How could I then justify eating organic animal products just because they've had a supposedly ok life? How is a dog any different to a lamb, a cow or a pig? They all have in common that they are animals that can feel fear and pain, but also excitement and joy.

At the end of the day, for every animal product, be it cheese or leather, a healthy animal has had to die prematurely for that product to exist.

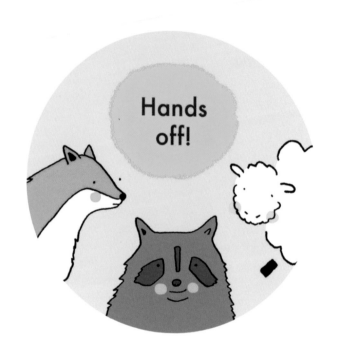

WHY NOT TO
WEAR ANIMALS

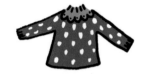

Being vegan means that we don't use animal products because they are not ours to take; they belong to the animal.

However, we live in a non-vegan world, so using animal products has been normalised and the extent of animal suffering is not widely known. A common misconception about animal products such as leather and wool is that they are a byproduct of the meat industry and consequently it is in a way better to use up resources that are already there. However, this for the most part is not true, and even when it is a "byproduct" there are still reasons why it is not ethical to purchase these animal products.

In the following section we will cover wool, leather, down, silk and fur.

WOOL

During a sheep's lifetime they suffer a lot. After a certain age a sheep's production of wool slows down, so they are no longer deemed profitable and are sent to be slaughtered for their meat and skin.

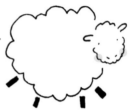

At the end of their lives they often have to travel very far and in horrible conditions.

Sheep that haven't been bred for the wool industry produce just enough wool to keep warm and shed any excess. However, commercial sheep have been bred so that they have wrinkly skin, which means higher production of wool and an inability to shed.

When sheep can't shed, flies can lay eggs between the folds of their skin, and once the maggots hatch the sheep's skin can be eaten. As a preventative measure farmers can perform a method called Mulesing, which involves cutting large strips of skin from the sheep without any anaesthesia, which is incredibly painful.

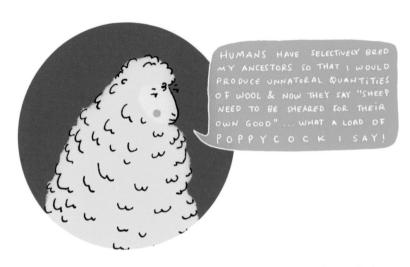

To obtain the wool sheep need to be sheared, and this is often done with force and pain. Workers are normally paid not by the hour but by volume. This means that the sheep is pinned down and shearing is rushed, with sheep often getting nicked or have pieces of flesh completely cut off. Shearing is done in the spring time just before the sheep would naturally shed their wool. This is because shearing later would result in a loss in wool harvest, so sheep are exposed to the elements too early on in the spring and can die.

Moreover, other practices such as tail-docking, castration and ear tagging are performed without anaesthesia, just as it is performed in the meat industry. Sheep in the wool industry are essentially factory farmed and the conditions that they live in are cruel, simply to commodify their wool.

LEATHER

Every year, more than a billion animals are killed for their flesh and skin. Leather is the skin of an animal, so the animal has had to die for a human to wear their skin. Sometimes there is the assumption that leather is a byproduct of the meat industry and consequently is not driving the market. However, this is not the case. Leather creates more profit per weight of animal than their flesh does, so leather is helping the meat industry be profitable. Cows are forced to endure castration, branding and de-horning without anaesthesia. Moreover, a lot of the leather sold comes from animals who are primarily slaughtered for their skins. So by purchasing leather you are supporting the meat industry.

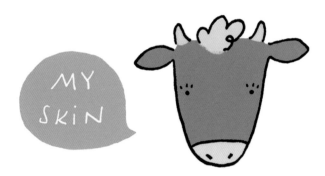

FUR

Fur is the hair of an animal that is still attached to their skin. Below are some of the animals that are killed for their fur:

MINK, DOGS, FOXES, RABBITS, RACCOONS, BEARS, CHINCHILLAS, CATS & MANY MORE.

Sometimes it comes from a fur farm, where the animals spend their short lives suffering in cramped, unhygienic cages. They are killed in various ways such as suffocation, electrocution, gassing, poisoning or drowning.

Alternatively animals are trapped in the wild, where they lay suffering from their wounds and the exposure to the cold, rain and wind.

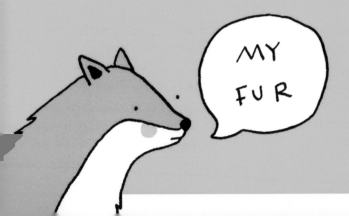

DOWN FEATHERS

Down can be found in some puffy jackets, pillows and bedding. Down is the soft feathers that are closest to the bird's skin. Sometimes it is plucked once the bird has been killed, but it is often obtained from live birds. The foie gras and poultry industries are also supported by the money made from selling down.

MY FLUFFLINESS IS MINE & NOT FOR YOU TO PLUCK FROM ME.

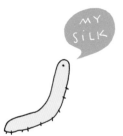

MY SILK

SILK

Silk is the material that silkworms make to wrap themselves in a cocoon. To harvest the silk the worms in their silk cocoons are boiled alive.

CONCLUSION

In any situation where humans try to profit off of animals, the animals' wellbeing is always compromised. Every pound we spend is a vote for the world we want to live in, so if we stop supporting markets that exploit animals, over time the market will shift towards more compassionate consumerism. Later on in the book, we will cover how to dress ethically easily and on a budget.

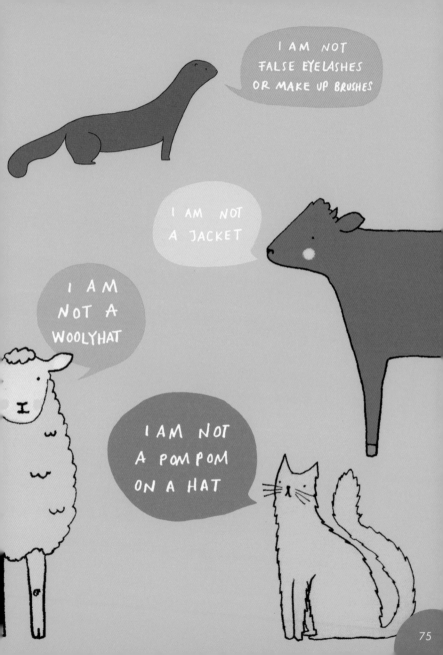

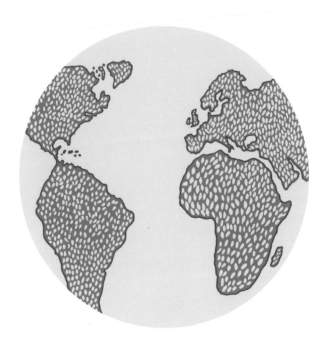

OUR PLANET

Our planet is our home. Your house/flat/boat, wherever you may live, provides you with shelter, warmth, somewhere to make food, somewhere to relieve yourself, running water and also enjoyment. Wherever you live right now most likely won't be the place that you will live forever, and, even if you do, once you die it won't be yours any longer. In a way you are a passing guest in your home, just like we are on planet Earth.

The planet does a lot for us that doesn't just happen by magic. Plants make it possible for us to breathe, the atmosphere is just right to keep us from boiling alive or turning into popsicles, we have fertile soil to grow food that nourishes us. These are called ecosystem services. We often take them for granted but we really shouldn't!

For the sake of self preservation, we should look after both our homes and our planet as much as possible. For example, if there was a gas leak in our home, we wouldn't just open a window and carry on; no, we would turn off the gas and fix the root of the problem. Animal agriculture is a massive contributor to climate change and environmental degradation, so it makes sense to not only have shorter showers, turn off lights and use the car less, but also to reduce our reliance on animal agriculture which is a major contributor.

In the following chapter we will be covering why becoming vegan is good for the planet and, consequently, good for the human race.

Animal agriculture has a detrimental impact on the planet. Animal products make up 56% to 58% of total agricultural greenhouse gases, despite only providing 37% of our protein and 18% of our calories globally. The impact can be broken down into three categories: resources consumed, outputs and disruption of environment.

RESOURCES IT CONSUMES

The major resources that animal agriculture uses are water, land and grain. However, it also uses other resources such as petrol for the transportation of animals, antibiotics and, in the case of fish farms, they use fish as feed. In the Amazon, cattle ranching is the primary reason for deforestation. The rainforest is being cut down at the rate of a football field every second. One of the main reasons for this is to make room for grazing cattle, but also to grow crops like soy to feed livestock such as cows, chickens, pigs and fish. Worldwide, 90% of soy is going to livestock. As well as water and land, more resources are needed to grow the feed, including pesticides and fertilisers which are used excessively. In most cases, soy is farmed intensively, so not only are ridiculous amounts of rainforest cut down to grow it, it also drains the soil without giving it a chance to recharge. That is when we see land degradation happen. From bio-diverse rainforests to crops to grass and, finally, to barren land. Water, a precious resource, is used abundantly to raise livestock and to grow their food.

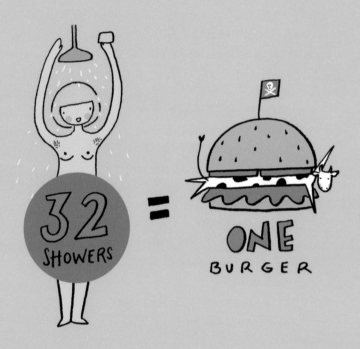

The water required to produce a beef burger is equivalent to 32 showers!

OUTPUTS

Methane is roughly 30 times more potent than carbon dioxide, and methane is what cows fart. Animal agriculture is directly responsible for 18% of all greenhouse gases, which is more than all transportation put together. Including deforestation and land use change, livestock is responsible for 30% of greenhouse gas emissions. A farm with 2500 dairy cattle produces a similar amount of waste as a city of 411,000 people. That means cows produce about 160 times more excrement than the humans! And unlike human excrement, it doesn't have drains that take it away to be treated. In the US alone livestock are responsible for roughly 55% of erosion, 37% of pesticides used, 50% of volume of antibiotics consumed, 32% of nitrogen load and 33% of the phosphorous load into freshwater sources. Excrement, urine, pesticides and fertilisers (used to grow the feed crops) are combined together and produced in huge volumes, so it is no wonder that animal agriculture is a massive contributor to ocean "dead zones".

Nitrous oxide is a greenhouse gas that is 296 times more warming than CO_2, and livestock is responsible for 65% of emissions. Livestock's contribution to CO_2 is 9% and for methane it's 37%. Livestock is responsible for 64% of anthropogenic ammonia emissions. Ammonia pollution can cause acid rain and acidification of ecosystems.

POOP

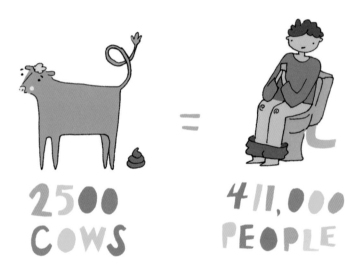

2500 COWS = **411,000 PEOPLE**

A farm of 2500 cows produces the same amount of poo as a city of 411,000 people!

DISRUPTION OF ENVIRONMENT

Animal agriculture is the leading cause of species extinction and habitat destruction. This is due to the amount of rainforest that has been cleared for livestock as well as the outputs from livestock. Livestock account for 20% of total terrestrial animal biomass and take up space that was once a habitat for wildlife. Marine ecosystems are also greatly affected due to the water pollution and ammonia emissions from livestock, as well as overfishing for feed.

EFFICIENCY

It doesn't make sense to feed millions of tonnes of crops such as soya to livestock when the livestock will create waste, disrupt the environment and, once sold, provide fewer calories than consumed. High-impact beef producers can create 105kg of CO_2 equivalents and use 370m^2 of land per 100 grams of protein, and low-impact beef producers can create from 8.7kg of CO_2 equivalents and use 7.4m^2. Compared to low-impact beans, peas and other plant-based proteins which can create just 0.3kg of CO_2 equivalents and use only 1m^2 of land for the same 100 grams of protein, including processing, packaging and transporting. The same study that provided the above results concluded that diets free of animal products deliver greater environmental benefits than purchasing sustainable meat or dairy. Even a low-impact litre of cow's milk uses nearly twice the amount of land and creates almost double the emissions of an average litre of soy milk. The study also showed that plant-based diets reduce food emissions by up to 73%, which not only includes greenhouse gases but also other emissions that degrade terrestrial and aquatic ecosystems. Additionally, without animal agriculture, we would require roughly 7.1 billion fewer hectares of farmland.

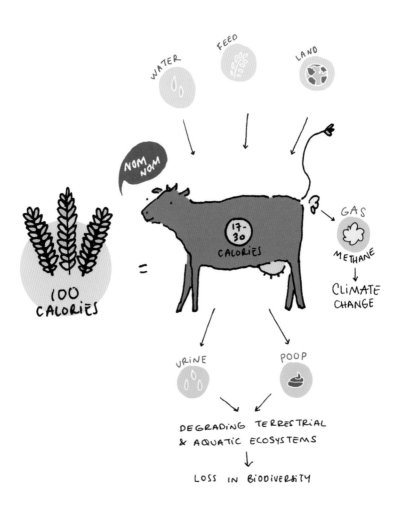

100 calories of grain are turned into 17 to 30 calories of meat. This is not an efficient way of feeding the world.

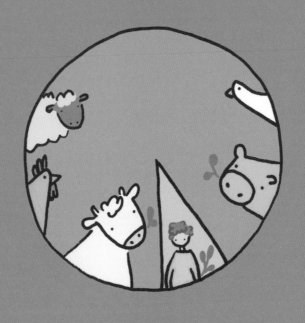

90% OF SOY
IS GOING
TO LIVESTOCK

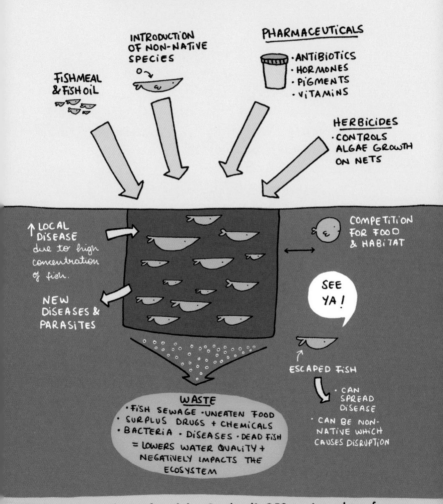

IMPACTS OF MARINE AQUACULTURE

INTRODUCTION OF NON-NATIVE SPECIES

PHARMACEUTICALS
- ANTIBIOTICS
- HORMONES
- PIGMENTS
- VITAMINS

FISHMEAL & FISH OIL

HERBICIDES
- CONTROLS ALGAE GROWTH ON NETS

↑ LOCAL DISEASE due to high concentration of fish.

COMPETITION FOR FOOD & HABITAT

NEW DISEASES & PARASITES

SEE YA!

ESCAPED FISH
- CAN SPREAD DISEASE
- CAN BE NON-NATIVE WHICH CAUSES DISRUPTION

WASTE
- FISH SEWAGE · UNEATEN FOOD
- SURPLUS DRUGS + CHEMICALS
- BACTERIA · DISEASES · DEAD FISH
= LOWERS WATER QUALITY + NEGATIVELY IMPACTS THE ECOSYSTEM

World Wide Fund once found that Scotland's 350 marine salmon farms produced more sewage waste in terms of nitrogen and phosphorus than the 5.1 million humans in Scotland.

IN CONCLUSION

This is what the current climate looks like. It is dire, and things get scarier when we add the fact that the global population is growing and people are increasing their consumption of animal products as they become more affluent. A change has to happen and it has to happen soon. A paper published in 2018 stated that transitioning towards more plant-based diets could reduce food related greenhouse gas emissions by up to 73%. Dietary shifts can help with our climate change mitigation plans, which need to be put in place before 2030 if we are to prevent further mass extinction, drought, flooding and devastation. The IPCC 2018 report states that not only can this shift contribute to reducing emissions but also would offer co-benefits such as improved access to drinking water, better health and the re-forestation of previously-farmed land.

NO OTHER CHANGE IN LIFESTYLE CAN HAVE AS BIG AN IMPACT

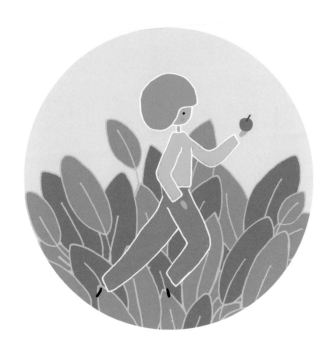

HEALTH

A vegan diet can provide all the neccesary nutrients that our body needs and can meet healthy eating guidelines.

Many people choose a vegan diet solely for the health benefits as some research has shown that it can have a positive effect on people's health in the short and long term.

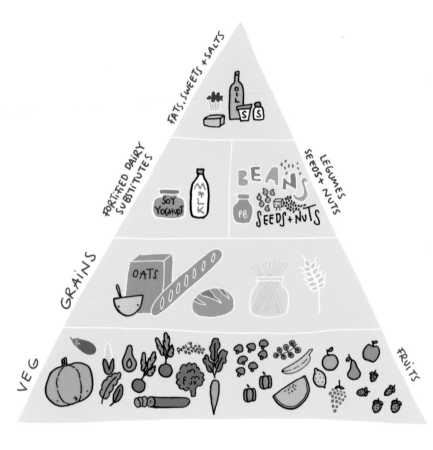

FATS, SWEETS + SALTS

FORTIFIED DAIRY SUBSTITUTES

LEGUMES SEEDS + NUTS

GRAINS

VEG

FRUITS

OIL

S S

SOY YOGHURT

M*LK

BEANS

PB

SEEDS + NUTS

OATS

PEAS

EAT THE RAINBOW!

Not all vegan diets are created equal! Vegans can be healthy and they can be unhealthy, so simply eating a vegan diet isn't going to magically give you unicorn powers. However, there have been many studies that show that eating a whole-foods, plant-based diet can have a wide range of health benefits.

So what is a whole-foods, plant-based diet?

It is a diet full of vegetables, whole grains, legumes, nuts and seeds, and low in processed sugar, oils and processed foods such as doughnuts, crisps and white flour.

80% of the antibiotics that are made in the US are sold to the animal industry.

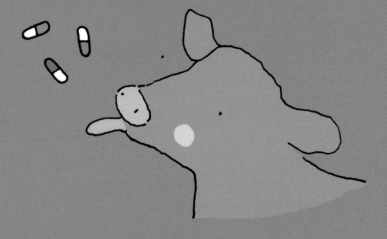

Why is a whole-foods, plant-based diet (WFPBD) good for you?

This is because animal products are replaced with veg, fruit, whole grains, pulses, seeds and nuts, which are high in vitamins, minerals and fibre.

By consuming calories from these sources, you are reducing your risk of health problems linked to diets high in animal products - such as type 2 diabetes, cancer, heart disease and other chronic illnesses.

Type 2 diabetes
A single egg a week can increase your chances of developing type 2 diabetes by 76%, 2 eggs a week doubles your odds and an egg a day triples the odds. Animal-based iron has also been found to increase the risk of type 2 diabetes, as well as fish consumption. This may be due to the omega-3 and also the contaminants that build up in fish.

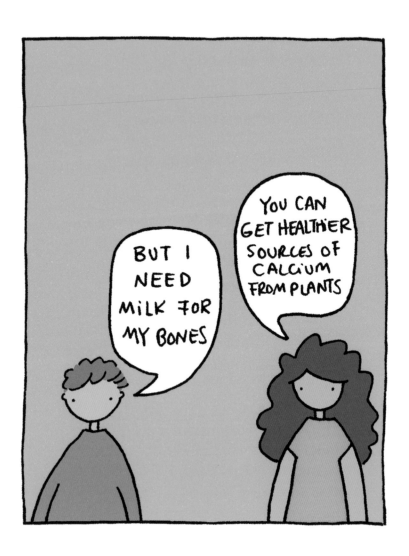

Cancers

Eggs are high in cholesterol, which aids malignant cells to rapidly grow and proliferate. Additionally they are high in animal protein and choline, which have been linked to increase risk of some cancers. Cohort studies show that consumption of dairy products were associated with increased risk of some cancers, partly due to the milk protein casein and whey, which helps prostate cancer cells to grow. Milk consumption has also been linked with higher risk of hip fracture.

Heart disease

Animal products are high in cholesterol and fat, which are linked to heart disease and make it harder for our bodies to heal. By adopting a balanced whole-foods, plant-based diet, you will help your body to heal because of the decrease in cholesterol and the increase of fibre. You'll also eliminate animal-based iron, which has been found to increase the risk of coronary heart disease, unlike plant-based iron.

Conclusion

Following a well balanced WFPBD can have a wide range of health benefits. As well as reducing risk of deadly cancers, some people experience more energy and better skin, and some vegan athletes claim to recover faster on a whole-foods, plant-based diet. To find out more, I would recommend reading the book How Not to Die by Michael Greger, M.D. Another recommended book is Becoming Vegan by nutritionist Brenda Davis.

My baby has to grow roughly 40 times faster than human babies and my milk makes that possible. But it's not designed for humans!

RECOMMENDED
DOCUMENTARIES

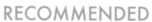

ANIMALS
Land of Hope and
   Glory
Earthlings
Rotten
Dominion
Speciesism: The Movie
Blackfish
The Ghost in Our
   Machine

ENVIRONMENT
Cowspiracy
More Than Honey
Meat The Truth
Before The Flood
H.O.P.E. What You
   Eat Matters

HEALTH
Food, Inc.
The Game Changers
Forks Over Knives
What the Health
Food Choices
Eating You Alive
Plantpure Nation

INSPIRATIONAL
73 Cows
Vegucated
Running For Good
Carnage
Vegan: Everyday
   Stories
Called to Rescue
Live and Let Live
Peaceable Kingdom
Vegan 2017

We have covered a lot, from animals to health to the environment. The point of showing you many different reasons why to be vegan is because we are all different, and what will motivate one person might not motivate someone else.

Even if you already have your *why*, it is important to be aware of the other reasons why to be vegan because we live in a non-vegan world and your way of living will be challenged by other people – and even yourself. Knowing all the facts about veganism can help you stay vegan. For me, I originally went vegan for the animals, but now I do it for a multitude of reasons. There are other reasons why to be vegan, such as the fact that slaughterhouse workers have among the highest rates of PTSD, depression and anxiety. Knowing the different reasons why to be vegan is important because, if one of them is challenged, then you've got more motivations rather than just one.

For example, if you've started your vegan journey for health reasons, and that is your only motivation, then there might be days where you think, "Well, I don't really care about my health today", and your vegan intentions might falter. However, if you have other reasons why to be vegan, it will be easier to keep yourself motivated.

There a lot of horrible facts and statistics about the animal agriculture sector. I don't tell you these to scare you but simply for you to be aware of them. For so long I didn't know that these things went on and I wish I had known earlier.

I hope the information has provided you with food for thought and has cemented your intentions of going vegan and/or staying vegan.

PART 2

How To Go Vegan

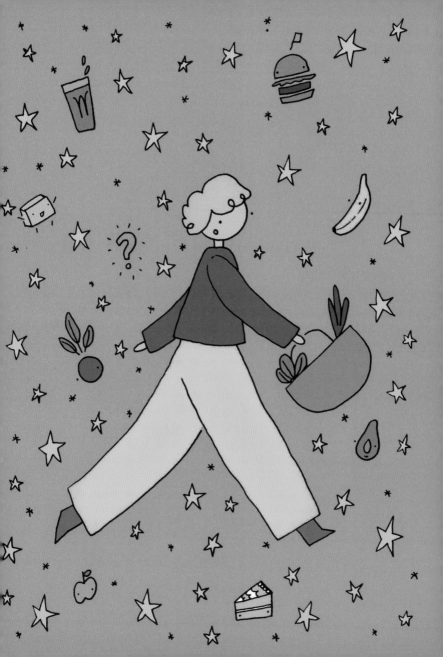

HOW TO GO VEGAN

You have now read all the evidence for why going vegan is good for the animals, for our planet and for your health.

So now you might be thinking:

"How do I go vegan and stay vegan!?"

We will cover common vegan myths, how to transition, how to eat vegan, where to get all your nutrients from and buying food and drinks. Read on for lots of information and tips on how to eat and drink as a vegan!

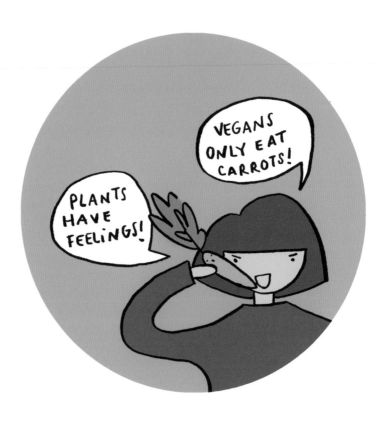

MYTHS + FAQ

Before we get started with how to transition and information on making your transition as easy and fun as possible, I think it is important that we start off with a clean slate. By that I mean that we should dispel and answer the most common myths and FAQs about veganism that might hinder your good intentions of going vegan.

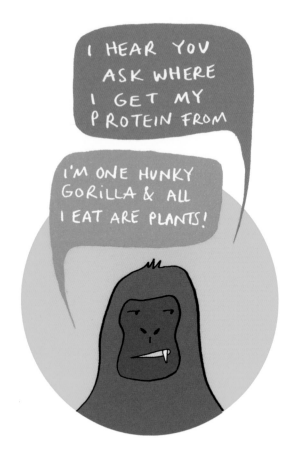

Humans need to eat meat to get protein.
Plants contain protein, which is where many animals get it from. By eating plant protein, you are eliminating the middleman and getting it straight from the source, while also bypassing cholesterol, antibiotics and a lot of other nasties. Simply put: If you are meeting your daily calorie requirements, this means that you are meeting your protein requirements.

Humans have canine teeth, therefore they are meant to eat animals.
The largest canine teeth belonging to a land mammal are those of the hippopotamus, which are herbivores. Their canines are much larger that those of lions and tigers! Gorillas also have large canines and are herbivores; they have them so as to tear and open fruits and plants. And even if our tiny human canines could rip through the tough flesh of an animal, how can we justify the death and suffering of an animal when, scientifically speaking, we can thrive on a vegan diet. Just because we have fists doesn't mean that we have to be violent.

Being vegan is expensive
When some people go vegan it's like discovering a new world full of yummy foods, so you can end up spending more money at first because you are eating out more or buying fancy vegan things. But take a look at what a vegan diet consists of: pulses such as beans and lentils, grains such as rice, bread and pasta, veggies and nuts. The first three groups are the cheapest foods you can find in a supermarket. Nuts can be a little expensive, but you don't have to go overboard with them to get the nutrients that you need. Ultimately a vegan diet can be much cheaper than buying meat and much healthier; however, like with any other foods, you can spend as little or as much as you'd like.

Top tip: search phrases like 'vegan on a budget' and hundreds of blogs, Facebook groups and YouTube videos will appear with local tips – there are also lots of useful websites and apps on pages 220-1 of this book.

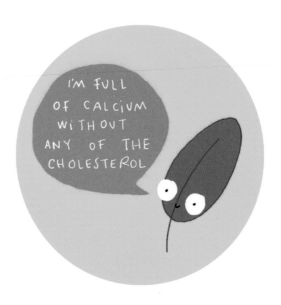

We need to drink milk for calcium

Humans are the only species to drink the milk of another species through adulthood. Lactose intolerance exists because we aren't designed to digest non-human breast milk. In fact, cultures that historically have drunk very little milk are very healthy and are not calcium-deficient at all. This is because plants such as broccoli and almonds have calcium. Not only that, but studies have shown that cow's milk can actually cause calcium to leach from our bones and can lead to osteoporosis. Milk also contains the protein casein, which is a carcinogen that promotes the growth of cancer cells.

Vegan food is boring

Vegan food, just like omni food, can come in all varieties, from boring to amazing. If you simply remove the animal products that you have been used to all your life and don't replace them with new foods, then, yes, it might be boring, and you might not be getting your calorific daily requirements. Replace them with high-energy foods such as chickpeas and tofu or any other legume. Learn new recipes and get excited about a whole new world of delicious food!

Vegans are unhealthy

There are unhealthy vegans and super healthy vegans and everything in between. It's really your decision of where you want to be. You could eat nothing but crisps and you would be unhealthy, or you could eat a whole-foods vegan diet and get all the nutrients and minerals that your body needs to flourish. Check out the Health section to find out more about how a vegan diet can actually make you a lot healthier.

Being vegan is extreme

Before becoming vegan I thought vegans were extreme. I admired vegetarians, but I didn't see what was wrong with milk, and I didn't know that male chicks in the egg industry get ground up or gassed alive, so I thought being vegan was unnecessary. After finding out how easy it could be to eat vegan – and finding out that dairy cows get separated from their babies so that we can drink their breast milk, and the mothers were killed at 4 years old instead living their full 25 years, and that if their baby is a boy it gets killed for veal – eating vegetables instead of animal products suddenly seemed a whole lot less extreme.

Vegans are... extreme, animal lovers, privileged, hippy, skinny, fat, preachy, loving, unhealthy, etc. Vegans come in all shapes and forms. Social media and the media in general tend to homogenise and create stereotypes of everything, and that includes what veganism looks like. But don't let beliefs or expectations that you might have of vegans deter you from your vegan journey. At the end of the day, you are still you, and you decide what that looks like.

Being vegan is hard

Being vegan shouldn't be hard because its just eating plants! However, we live in a non-vegan world, so there is a learning curve to being vegan, from reading labels to looking up whether that beer is vegan. But like with all learning curves, you reach the top and it's pretty chill afterwards because you have all this knowledge and experience that you didn't have before. Whenever people ask me if being vegan is hard, I can honestly say that it isn't, but I do remember sometimes feeling a bit overwhelmed with reading labels and wondering, AM I GETTING ENOUGH PROTEIN? at the beginning of my vegan journey. I didn't transition over night and this helped me to learn along the way without feeling too overwhelmed. Privilege also comes into play here, as some people will have easier access to fresh fruit and veg, more time or money than others and all sorts of other factors. But what matters is that you are here and you are on your way.

IT GETS EASIER!

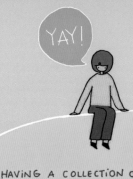

HOW TO GO VEGAN

Now that we have covered the reasons for going vegan and busted some myths about veganism that might have hindered your transition, we can get onto how to actually transition!

There are two ways of transitioning, over night or gradually.

You might choose to transition over night if you feel like you already have done quite a bit of research on why to go vegan, what foods you might eat and feel equipped to embark on your vegan life.

A more gradual transition has the benefit of allowing more time for you to cut out animal products and get used to cooking vegan meals. This might be more suited for people who find that if they fall off the wagon they stay off the wagon. In other words, if you know yourself and overnight transitioning is not for you and you feel that a gradual transition might be more sustainable, then go for it! It can also be better to change gradually if your diet before consisted mostly of animal products, as a sudden drastic change in diet can take your body by surprise.

Both routes are equally valid, and both routes have their pros and cons. It is more down to you as an individual to determine which will work best for you.

BE KIND

Being kind to yourself is the most important thing to remember, both whilst transitioning and after being vegan

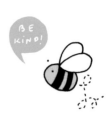

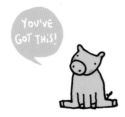

Yes, you might experience guilt if you accidentally ate something non-vegan or slipped up, especially if your main motivation is the animals.

But there is a point where perfectionism might make you feel like you failed at being vegan, so to protect yourself from feeling like a failure you might decide to just give up on.

But trying and failing is sometimes better overall than not trying at all. Veganism is about compassion for all animals, and humans are animals after all. So practice compassion towards other fellow humans and yourself.

OVER NIGHT

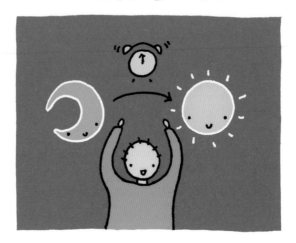

Transitioning over night
If you prefer to rip the band aid right off then I would
recommend watching as many documentaries as
possible. Some are graphic, others are not; however,
there is value in the graphic footage because for so long
we have been conditioned to believe that animals
farmed for food lead happy lives, and the ignorance of
the animals' pain has allowed us to carry on with our
choices.
Make a list of all the vegan meals that you can make
and join your local online vegan group to find out where
to find yummy vegan food. Set a date of when you want
to go vegan over night and enter that day with
excitement and a sense of adventure!

SLOW & STEADY

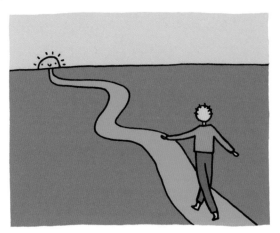

Gradual transition

The tips are mostly similar to those above, but with the difference that you are doing things gradually. So you might either set dates to quit one animal product at a time, or you might be more open ended in that you watch documentaries, read up on veganism, cook more veganised meals. Over time you will find that you don't even want to eat certain animal products because they no longer appeal to you.

Resources to help you transition
- Challenge22
- VeGuide app by The Vegan Society
- 31 Day Vegan Pledge by Veganuary

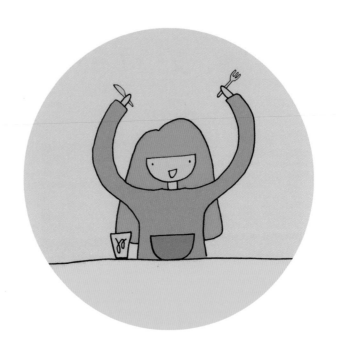

WHAT VEGANS
EAT IN A DAY

There are literally endless possibilities of
what you can eat as a vegan! The
following pages are filled with examples
of different things you can eat as a vegan
for breakfast, lunch, dinner, snacks and
dessert to get you inspired!

BREAKFAST

SMOOTHIE BOWL

TOFU SCRAMBLE

PORRIDGE
OPTIONS:
BANANAS
FROZEN FRUIT
MAPLE SYRUP
COCONUT FLAKES
CINNAMON

CHICKPEA FLOUR OMELETTE WITH VEG
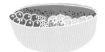

CEREAL / GRANOLA

MUSHROOMS ON TOAST

OAT M*LK

WAFFLES & FRUIT

CHEEZE TOASTIE

AVOCADO + HUMMOS ON TOAST

HOT CHOC COFFEE TEA

SMOOTHIE

PANCAKES

FULL ON BREAKFAST
• HASH BROWNS
• VEGGIE SAUSAGES
• BEANS
• TOFU SCRAMBLE
• TOMATOES
• MUSHROOMS.

SPREAD ON YOUR TOAST!
      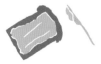

WHOLE EARTH   CHOC   JAM   MARMITE   VEGO

LUNCH

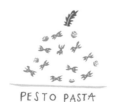

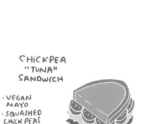

PESTO PASTA

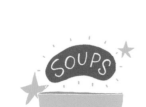

CHICKPEA
"TUNA"
SANDWICH

· VEGAN
  MAYO
· SQUASHED
  CHICKPEAS
· AVO (OPTIONAL)
· LETTUCE
· TOMATOES

SOUPS

PESTO PASTA

TOFU SCRAMBLE

PASTA WITH HUMMUS
CHICKPEAS AND VEGGIES

BURRITO WITH BEANS,
VEGGIES AND RICE

QUORN FISH-LESS FINGER
SANDWICH

ASIAN NOODLE BOWL WITH
GINGER & PEANUT DRESSING

SOUPS
(LENTIL - TOMATO - PEA &
COURGETTE - LEEK & POTATO -
CARROT - MISO)

VEGAN CRAB CAKES & SALAD

PULLED JACKFRUIT WRAP

DiNNER

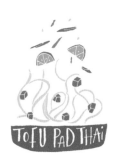

TOFU PAD THAI

VEGAN LASAGNE (USING A BECHAMEL MADE WITH OIL, PLANT MILK AND FLOUR, OR BLENDING WHITE BEANS WITH NUTRITIONAL YEAST)

"TUNA" BAKE (USING CHICKPEAS; AND NORI SHEETS TO GET THE TUNA TASTE)

CHILLI SIN CARNE

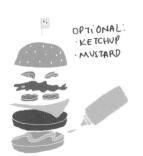

OPTIONAL:
· KETCHUP
· MUSTARD

VEGAN BURGER USING LINDA McCARTNEY PATTIES

TOFU, MUSHROOM & SPINACH QUICHE

PAELLA, USING CHICKPEAS INSTEAD OR FRY'S "CHICKEN"

SPAGHETTI BOLOGNESE (USING VEGAN MINCE OR GENTLY PULSE MUSHROOMS)

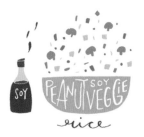

SOY

PEANUT SOY VEGGIE rice

PIZZA - THE NEAPOLITAN WAY (WITHOUT CHEESE) OR WITH VEGAN CHEEZE

SNACKS

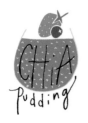

CHIA PUDDING

TOAST WITH BANANA + NUT BUTTER

PLANT YOGHURT + FRUIT + NUTS

DATES OR FIGS

ROASTED CHICKPEAS

FRUIT + PEANUT BUTTER

GUACAMOLE + VEG

NUTS

HUMMUS + VEGGIES

HOME-MADE KALE CHIPS

PITA + VEGAN TZATZIKI

GRANOLA BARS

RICE CAKES + NUT BUTTERS

DESSERTS

All of your favourite desserts can be made vegan! Check out the sections on dairy replacements and vegan baking, plus the Resources pages, for inspiration!

CHOCOLATE CHIP BANANA BREAD

APPLE CRUMBLE

SCONES

CUPCAKES/MUFFINS

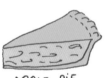

APPLE PIE

DOUBLE CHOCOLATE CHIP COOKIES

MERINGUE PIE

RASPBERRY TARTLETS

BROWNIE & ICE CREAM

CHOCOLATE MOUSSE

DOUGHNUTS

MUG CAKES - CAKE FOR ONE MADE IN THE MICROWAVE!

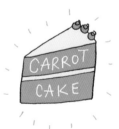

CHEESECAKE

LEARNING NEW RECIPES

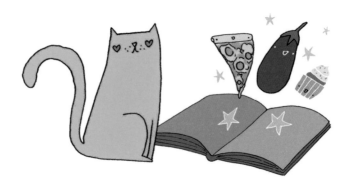

Getting new vegan recipes under your belt will make the transition so much easier and yummier! You can learn new recipes through a variety of ways.

It's simple to use the internet to find amazing resources, such as food blogs and vegan websites. YouTube is great for finding videos of people sharing meal preps and recipes of what they eat in a day as a vegan, from the quick, easy and cheap meal preps to more complex recipes such as homemade seitan "chicken" nuggets!

To find the recipes that will make your vegan transition easier and more fun, it is also important to get inspired!

VEGANISE

Veganising your favourite meals that you used to enjoy as an omni is a great place to start if you're feeling a bit lost for what to cook.

iT!

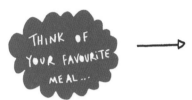

THINK OF YOUR FAVOURITE MEAL...

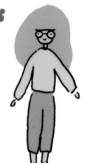

SEARCH

VEGAN LASAGNA RECIPE 🔍

GET COOKING!

EXAMPLES:

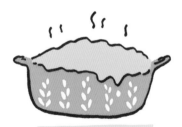

SHEPHERD'S PIE

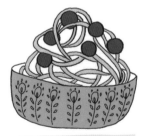

SPAGHETTI BOLOGNESE

GET INSPIRED

An important step in your vegan journey is to get inspired and get excited! This will ensure that going vegan isn't something you see as limiting or difficult to maintain.

There are many sources of inspiration covered in the following pages.

The internet has a wealth of resources to get inspired. Try creating a Pinterest board of all the yummy vegan recipes that catch your eye, or make a YouTube playlist of videos that teach you step by step how achieve that perfect lasagne. Below are some of my favourite food YouTube accounts:

Pick Up Limes, Avant Garde Vegan, Peaceful Cuisine, SweetPotatoSoul, Edgy Veg, The Easy Vegan, The Vegan Corner, Cheap Lazy Vegan, Hot for Food, Unnatural Vegan

Searching through Instagram hashtags for vegan food can help you find amazing accounts with beautiful pictures of food and links to where to find the recipes.

If you are not a fan of the internet, then checking out your local library for their vegan recipe cookbooks and going out to vegan restaurants and cafes is a great way to explore what vegan food has to offer. Vegan festivals are also a great place to discover new food and not have to ask whether something is vegan!

Finally, getting together with friends to cook vegan food. Organising a pot lock is a cheap and easy way to try new recipes!

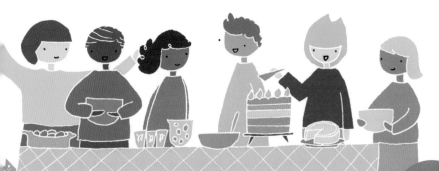

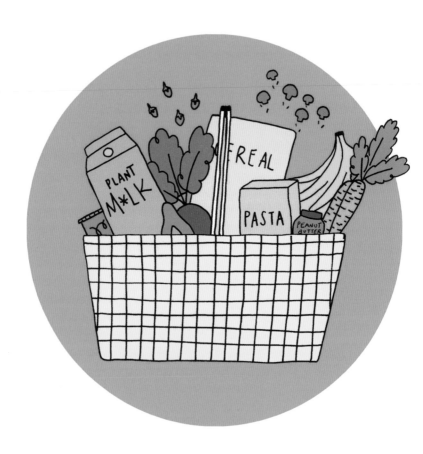

GROCERY
SHOPPING

When you first go vegan, a trip to the supermarket might seem daunting. You might think *but what can I even buy?* We humans have a negative bias, which means that we tend to predict the worst, especially in areas where we don't feel comfortable, but I'm here to tell you it is not that as hard as it might seem!

The following pages will prepare you for a straightforward shopping trip to stock up on delicious food.

CUPBOARD STAPLES

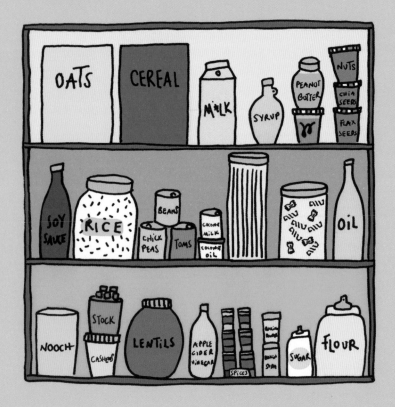

Once you go vegan you might panic and wonder what you will eat, but don't worry! Many items that you have in your cupboards are already vegan! But just in case you've moved into a new place and your cupboards are bare, here are some things to stock up on:

GRAINS (rice, quinoa, oats, couscous, millet, barley, farro) - **PASTA & NOODLES** (most are vegan) - **BEANS** (kidney, cannellini, black, baked) - **CHICKPEAS - LENTILS - TOFU - TOMATOES - COCONUT MILK - TAHINI**

PEANUT/ALMOND BUTTER - MOLASSES - DRIED FRUIT - OAT & FRUIT BARS - CEREAL - FLOUR - BAKING POWDER - BICARB - MAPLE SYRUP - BREAD - M*LK (oat, soy, hemp) - NUTS (almonds, cashews) SEEDS (flaxseed, chia, pumpkin)

SOY SAUCE - SRIRACHA - MISO - VEGETABLE STOCK - NUTRITIONAL YEAST - VINEGAR - OIL - HERBS & SPICES (chilli flakes/powder, basil, oregano, rosemary, thyme, cumin, onion powder, ginger)

Extras
LIQUID SMOKE - NORI SHEETS - VITAL WHEAT GLUTEN - CHICKPEA FLOUR - BLACK SALT (KALA NAMAK)

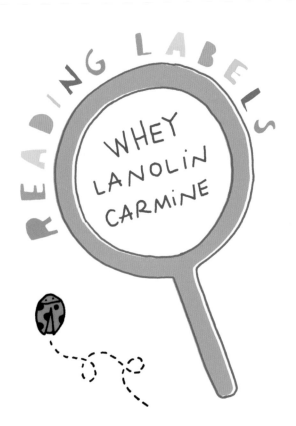

READING LABELS

WHEY
LANOLIN
CARMINE

Reading labels feels daunting at first, but I promise it becomes second nature!
Plus, more and more things are now being labelled VEGAN, which makes grocery shopping so much easier.

In the UK, most allergens such as **milk**, **eggs** and **fish** will be in bold, which makes reading labels easier, but sometimes they are listed under different forms such as whey and lactose. However, meat products won't always be in bold so, unless a product states it's vegetarian you should always be looking through all the ingredients.

Quite a lot of products are labelled vegetarian and a lot of them are actually vegan! Some common ingredients that will make a vegetarian product not vegan are milk, eggs, whey and casein. If these are not present then the product is most likely vegan. However, there are some more uncommon ingredients that might make an appearance, which we will cover on the next page.

When you find a product that seems vegan but it says "May contain milk", for example, it is still vegan. It just means that it was made in a factory where that allergen is present.

Some common non-vegan ingredients that originate from bones to crushed insects!

WHEY - from milk, and can be found in crisps and baked goods

LACTOSE - from milk

CASEIN - from milk

HONEY - produced by bees

ROYAL JELLY - worker bees ooze this substance to feed queens-to-be

VITAMIN D - from fish liver oil, unless it states it is D2 or that it is plant-based

ASPIC - (alternative to gelatine) jelly made from meat stock

LARD/TALLOW - animal fat

KERATIN - derived from skin, bones and connective tissues

PROPOLIS - collected by bees to build their hives

ALBUMEN/ALBUMIN - normally from eggs

PEPSIN - from the stomachs of pigs

SNEAKY E NUMBERS

E120 CARMINE - crushed and boiled beetles. Can be used as food colouring.

E441 GELATINE - obtained by boiling animal bones, skin and other bits. Found in chewy sweets, jelly, medicine capsules.

E542 BONE PHOSPHATE - ground up animal bones used as anti-caking agent, emulsifier and in some toothpastes.

E901 BEESWAX - wax secreted by bees to make their honeycombs. Used in shiny sweets and cosmetics.

E904 SHELLAC - made from a resin excreted by a female lac bug. Used as a glaze in sweets.

E910, E920, E921 L-CYSTEINE - made from animal hair and feathers. Used to speed up the commercial process of making breads, bagels and other doughs.

E913 LANOLIN - derived from wool. Used in cosmetics or to make vitamin D3.

E966 LACTITOL - sweetener derived from lactose, which is made from animal milk. Used as a synthetic sugar in low calorie foods.

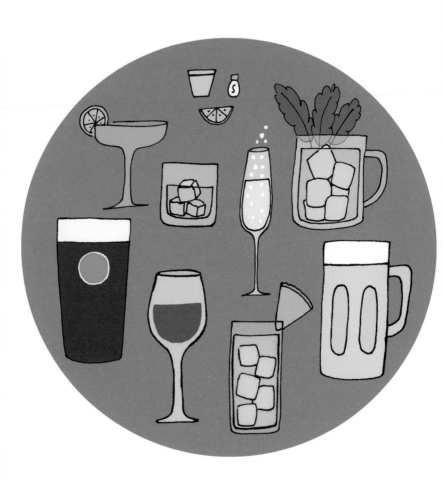

VEGAN
DRINKING

What do you drink as a vegan? It probably isn't the first thing that pops into your head because it might seem a bit strange that alcohol would contain animal products. However, they can be present in the ingredients, or are used in the filtering process. Dairy, honey and even meat can be ingredients in the final product, whilst isinglass (derived from fish bladders), gelatine, sea shells and egg whites are some of the products that can be used in the filtering process. Don't worry; there are plenty of beverages out there that do not use animal products in their filtration processes.

If a bottle is not labelled vegan or if you are unsure, Barnivore is handy website were you can type in the name of the alcohol and it will give you information on it. However, most of the time a quick search on the internet – such as "is Guinness vegan?" – will give you an answer quickly.
It is by the way!

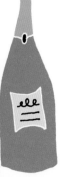

MILK ALTERNATIVES

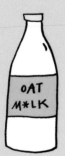

SOYA - OAT - RICE - ALMOND - BARLEY - CASHEW - COCONUT - PEA - PEANUT - HAZELNUT - HEMP

There are now dozens of different kinds of plant milks. Plant milk can be made from nuts, legumes or even seeds! With so many varieties, there is plant milk out there for everyone.

Some are sweet, some are nutty and some taste very similar to cows milk, but with none of the animal cruelty and cholesterol.

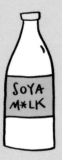

With veganism gaining momentum, plant milks are becoming more and more accessible and affordable. You can find them in the long life section in supermarkets, and most cafés offer soya milk at no extra cost!

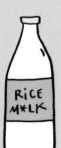

Oat, almond and cashew milk are the easiest to make at home, oat being the most sustainable and cheapest to make!

DAIRY ALTERNATIVES

ICE CREAM - CHEESE - DOUBLE CREAM -
CUSTARD - BUTTER - WHIPPED CREAM -
YOGURT - SOUR CREAM - MAYONNAISE

For every dairy product that you can think of there is a vegan alternative! There are many different varieties available to buy in larger supermarket. They range from supermarket own brands to artisan cheeses. Nowadays, more and more restaurants and cafés are offering these alternatives, so you don't have to miss out on cheezy pizza!

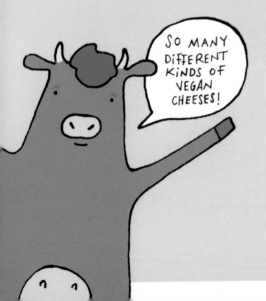

SO MANY DIFFERENT KINDS OF VEGAN CHEESES!

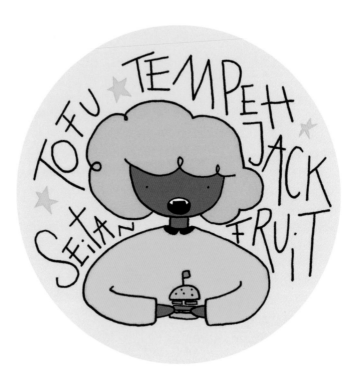

MEAT
ALTERNATIVES

MEAT ALTERNATIVES
The most well-known meat alternative is tofu; however, there are numerous meat alternatives in the market, and some you can even make yourself!

TOFU
You might have already tried tofu and thought "that's not for me!" But did you know that tofu comes in many different forms? From silky to extra firm, from tasteless to super flavoursome, it just depends on how it is prepared.

SEITAN
Also known as wheat gluten – as the name suggests, it is made from gluten in wheat. It originated in Asia and has been around for thousands of years. It is very similar to chicken in its texture, and you can even make it at home!

JACKFRUIT
Used in vegan "pulled pork" recipes thanks to its texture, jackfruit can be found in Asian supermarkets. Just make sure to get the type that is packed in brine and not the sweet one!

TEMPEH

Tempeh is made from fermented soya, so not only does it have the nutritional qualities of tofu but it is also a great probiotic.

VEGGIES AND LEGUMES

Some veggies, such as mushrooms, cauliflower or aubergine, when seasoned and cooked right can be a filling and tasty alternative to meat in a dish. Legumes can be great for making veggie burgers or even to make a shepherd's pie.

NO PREP MEAT ALTERNATIVES

Store-bought meat alternatives are especially great during your transition. The meat product I missed the most was chicken nuggets, but thankfully I found out about Fry's chicken nuggets, which are vegan, super yummy and very similar to what I remember chicken nuggets to taste like. Fry's Family Food do other vegan products as well. Other good brands to look out for are: Linda McCartney Foods, Tofurky, Vivera and Quorn, and lots of supermarkets are now doing their own line of vegan meats, such as Iceland. Not all of these brands are exclusively vegan, so make sure that it states "suitable for vegans".

WHY EAT ANIMALS

ANIMALS

WHEN THERE ARE ALTERNATIVES AVAILABLE?

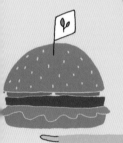

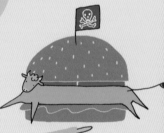

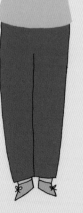

ONE EGG EQUALS

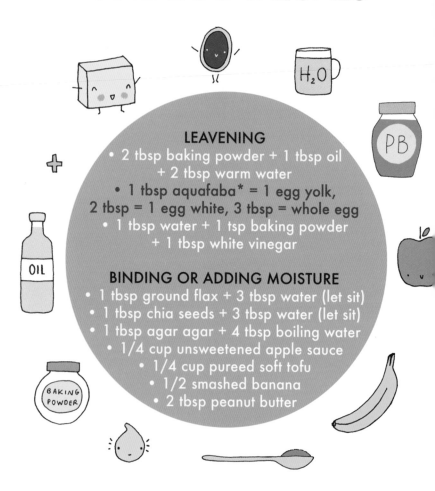

LEAVENING
- 2 tbsp baking powder + 1 tbsp oil + 2 tbsp warm water
- 1 tbsp aquafaba* = 1 egg yolk, 2 tbsp = 1 egg white, 3 tbsp = whole egg
- 1 tbsp water + 1 tsp baking powder + 1 tbsp white vinegar

BINDING OR ADDING MOISTURE
- 1 tbsp ground flax + 3 tbsp water (let sit)
- 1 tbsp chia seeds + 3 tbsp water (let sit)
- 1 tbsp agar agar + 4 tbsp boiling water
- 1/4 cup unsweetened apple sauce
- 1/4 cup pureed soft tofu
- 1/2 smashed banana
- 2 tbsp peanut butter

* Aquafaba is the viscous water that comes in canned beans and legumes. Chickpea water is the most commonly used. It can be whipped just like egg whites into stiff peaks. Very useful to make meringues!

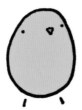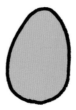

Eggs were the last thing that I found difficult to let go. However, once I made scrambled tofu, the taste and texture was so yummy that I no longer missed eggs!

All you need is firm tofu, onion, cumin powder, garlic powder, turmeric and a little water. Sauté the onion in a pan before crumbling in the tofu, adding the spices, a couple of table spoons of water and some cherry tomatoes. Allow some time for the flavours to infuse into the tofu. These go well on their own, on toast or as part of a full fry up! You can also add black salt which gives an eggy taste.

Chickpea flour is also a great ingredient to use in making vegan omelettes or quiches. There are also instant vegan products available where all you have to do is add water!

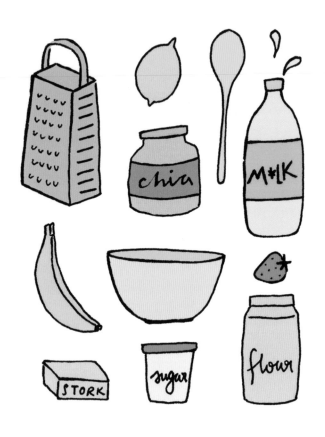

VEGAN
BAKING

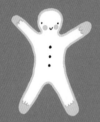

Maybe you used to be a keen baker or maybe you are new to baking in general. Either way you won't have to miss out on cakes and meringues just because you are now vegan!

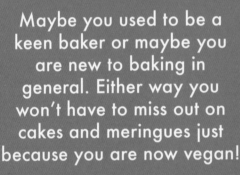

TOP TIP

With vegan baking it is essential that you don't over-mix your batter, otherwise you will end up with a dense cake.

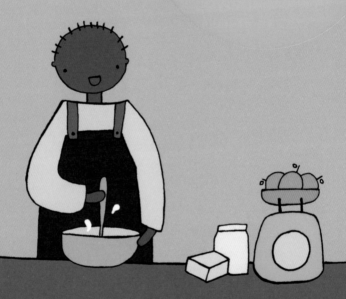

VEGAN BAKING TIPS

Before you dive into vegan baking, I would advise you to inspire yourself with fellow vegan bakers who have a bit of experience under their hat. There are many wonderful vegan baking blogs, YouTube accounts and cookbooks!

Vegan recipes will give their own instructions for replacing eggs, but on page 144 the most popular ones have been presented. The leavening replacements are for anything that needs to rise, like cakes.

Most sugar in the UK is vegan, but some are processed with bone char so do double check. When baking, make sure to not over-mix as this will lead to a dense cake. Mix just enough to incorporate the ingredients, but no more. Don't be afraid of a few lumps.

For quick, easy baking treats, Jus-rol do puff pastry, croissants, pain au chocolate and cinnamon rolls. All of which are vegan! Finally, microwave mug cakes are perfect for an impromptu cake for one!

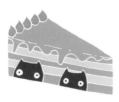

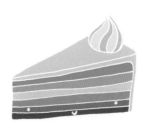

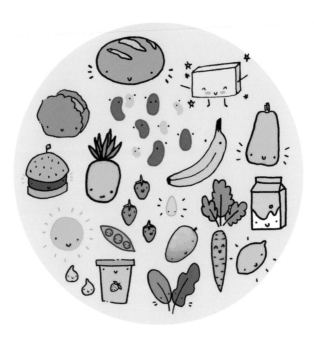

NUTRITION

The following pages are full of examples of where to get all your different vitamins and minerals. They aren't there so as to stress you out and obsess over what you're eating. Quite the opposite, they are there as a reassurance that you can get everything you need from a vegan diet. The key is to eat the rainbow, meaning a varied diet with lots of veggies, fruits, pulses and nuts.

It was only when I went vegan that I started stressing out about my health, partly because society has created the stereotype that if you are vegan you are either super healthy or super unhealthy. This binary way of thinking isn't helpful. Before I was vegan I rarely thought about whether I was getting all my requirements and nobody was asking me where I was getting my fibre from whilst I scoffed down a McDonalds. I could have done with thinking about what I ate a bit more back then. Now, if I could go back in time and give newly-vegan self advice, it would be to not stress so much and carry on eating my hummus.

VITAMIN A

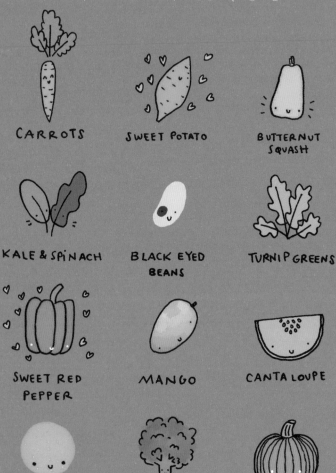

CARROTS

SWEET POTATO

BUTTERNUT SQUASH

KALE & SPINACH

BLACK EYED BEANS

TURNIP GREENS

SWEET RED PEPPER

MANGO

CANTALOUPE

GRAPEFRUIT

BROCCOLI

PUMPKIN

VITAMIN B

NUTRITIONAL YEAST

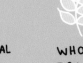

WHOLE GRAINS

NUTS

LEAFY GREENS

AVOCADO

MUSHROOMS

SEEDS

SWEET POTATO

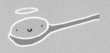

WHEAT GERM

FORTIFIED FOODS

PEAS

LEGUMES

VITAMIN B12

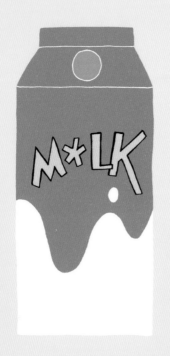

Fortified plant-based foods such as m*lks, cereals, nutritional yeast and others tend to have B12 added to them.

However, getting enough every day is very important, so supplementing with a B12 vitamin is a good idea.

VITAMIN C

ORANGES

PEPPERS

STRAWBERRIES

BLACK CURRANTS

BROCCOLI

PINEAPPLE

BRUSSELS SPROUTS

LEMON

CABBAGE

THYME

CAULIFLOWER

GRAPEFRUIT

VITAMIN D

Exposure to sunshine. Our bodies can create our own vitamin D!

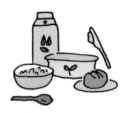

M*lks, breakfast cereals and spreads are usually fortified with vitamin D.

In colder climates it can be difficult to obtain vitamin D. So depending on how much sun you get, a supplement might be a good idea.

VITAMIN E

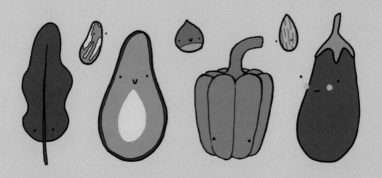

Leafy greens such as swish chard and spinach, avocados, red peppers, aubergine, parsnip, leek, Brazil nuts, hazelnuts, almonds, pine nuts, rye grain, quinoa, black beans, apricot, mango, peach and many more whole foods contain vitamin E.

VITAMIN K

Vitamin K can be found in broccoli and leafy greens such as kale, spinach, collards & swish chard. It can also be produced by our intestinal bacteria!

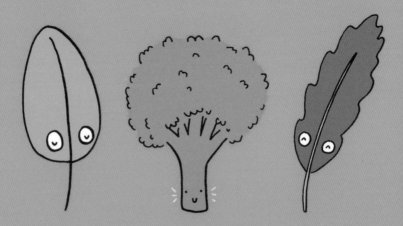

CALCIUM

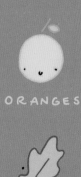

ORANGES

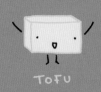

TOFU

WHITE BEANS

COLLARD GREENS

ALMONDS

SOY MILK

CHIA SEEDS

SOY YOGURT

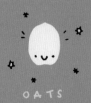

OATS

BLACK STRAP
MOLASSES

SESAME SEEDS

CHICKPEAS

PROTEIN

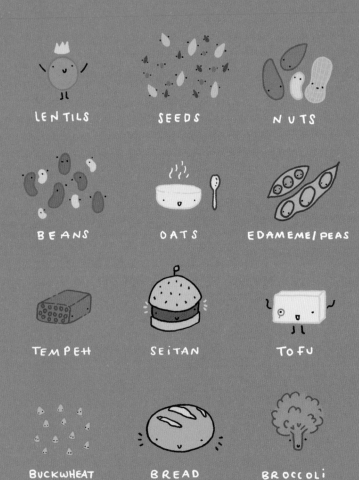

LENTILS

SEEDS

NUTS

BEANS

OATS

EDAMEME/PEAS

TEMPEH

SEITAN

TOFU

BUCKWHEAT

BREAD

BROCCOLI

IRON

LENTILS

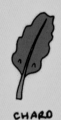

CHARD

MOLASSES

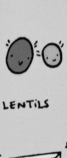

TOFU

RED KIDNEY
BEANS

POTATOES

PEAS

CHICKPEAS

SPINACH

OATS

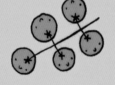

TOMATOES

MUSHROOM

ZINC

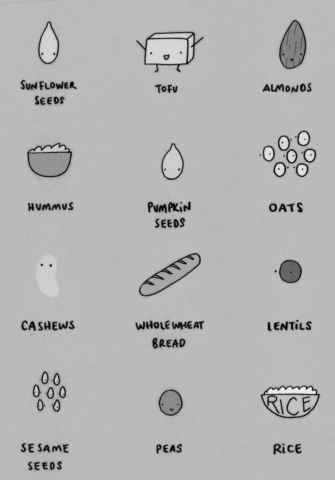

SUNFLOWER SEEDS

TOFU

ALMONDS

HUMMUS

PUMPKIN SEEDS

OATS

CASHEWS

WHOLE WHEAT BREAD

LENTILS

SESAME SEEDS

PEAS

RICE

MAGNESIUM

GREEN LEAFY VEGETABLES -
AVOCADOS - EDAMAME - CACAO
POWDER - PUMPKIN SEEDS - BLACK
BEANS - KIDNEY BEANS - SOYA BEANS
- SOY M*LK - ALMONDS - PEANUT
BUTTER - TAHINI - BRAZIL NUTS
CASHEWS - WHOLEGRAIN BREAD &
RICE - POTATOES - OATS - BANANAS

AND MANY MORE!

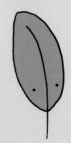
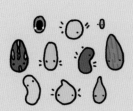
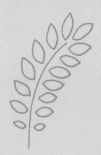

IODINE

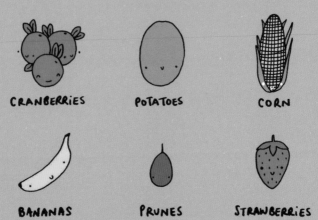

CRANBERRIES   POTATOES   CORN

BANANAS   PRUNES   STRAWBERRIES

Iodine is present in a lot of plant-based foods such as the ones listed above, and others such as green beans, green leafy vegetables, lima beans and even whole grains. However, the quantities vary depending on the soil that they are grown in.

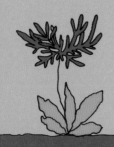

Sea vegetables can contain really high levels of iodine and so only a sprinkling of them is needed!

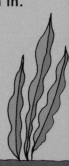

OMEGA 3 & 6

Ground flaxseeds - Flax seed oil - Olive oil - Nuts and nut oils such as walnuts and almonds - Tofu - Cooked soy beans - Soy oil - Canola oil - Chia seeds - Hemp seeds and Hemp oil - Tempeh

OiL

FIBRE

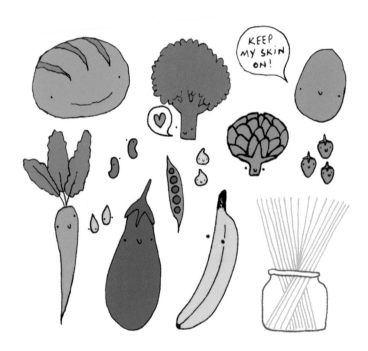

Fibre is super easy to get in a vegan diet!
Below are some of the foods that are high in fibre:

ALL FRUIT AND VEGETABLES -
WHOLE GRAINS SUCH AS OATS, SPELT &
WHEAT - NUTS & SEEDS - ALL BEANS & PULSES

CARBOHYDRATES

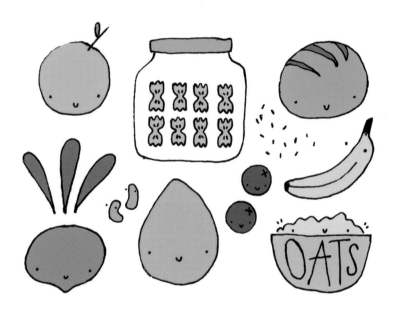

Carbohydrates often get a bad reputation, but complex carbs are great for keeping us full for longer and releasing energy throughout the day. However, simple carbs such as sugar should be avoided.

WHOLE GRAINS SUCH AS BROWN RICE, QUINOA, MILLET, BUCKWHEAT, OATS, WHEAT, BARLEY, SPELT - BEANS & PULSES - POTATOES - CEREALS - PASTA

PART 3

Living Vegan

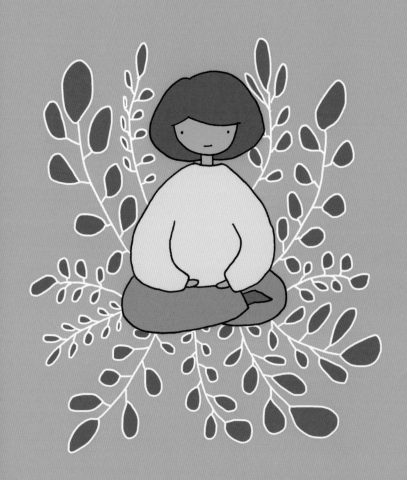

LIVING

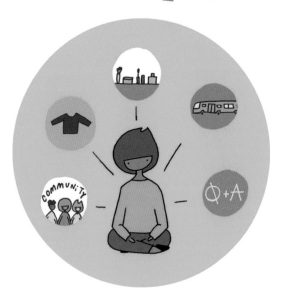

VEGAN

Veganism is so much more than just what we put in our mouths, it is how we live our lives.

Animal exploitation is present in every part of our lives, from the bathroom products we use to leather belts. But there's no need to worry: there are many alternatives and your way of living doesn't have to change drastically. Think of veganism as just another preference, like the ones you already have.

In the following chapter, we cover topics ranging from travelling tips to why zoos aren't vegan.

TOILETRIES & COSMETICS

There are two reasons why personal care products might not be vegan. They might be tested on animals and/or they might contain animal products as ingredients.

Animal testing

Animals like bunnies and puppies are often used in animal testing. They are forced to ingest the product being tested, such as shampoo or nail polish, until it kills them. Other tests involve placing the substance directly on animals' eyes to see the damage that it does. No one wants this, so look for the leaping bunny symbol for products not tested on animals.

Animal ingredients

Just because something is labelled as being 'cruelty-free' it doesn't necessarily mean that it doesn't contain animal products, so beware of this. Animal fat, beeswax and lanolin are some of the most common animal ingredients. There are plant-based alternatives for all of these. Isn't it nice to know that you are not lathering your face with bits of animals?

Animal parts

Some make-up brushes, false eyelashes and hair brushes use real animal hair, so it is important to keep this in mind when purchasing these items.

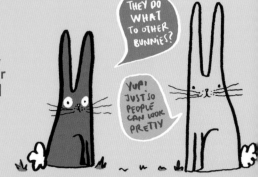

THEY DO WHAT TO OTHER BUNNIES?

YUP! JUST SO PEOPLE CAN LOOK PRETTY

ANIMAL INGREDIENTS

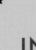

LANOLIN - derived from wool. Used as a moisturiser in creams and lip products.

COLLAGEN - from bones, skin and other parts of animals. Used in anti-ageing products.

ELASTIN - similar to collagen. Obtained from muscles and ligaments.

BONE PHOSPHATE - ground up animal bones used in some toothpastes.

SHELLAC - resin excreted by a female lac bug. Used in nail products and some hair sprays.

KERATIN - derived from skin, bones and connective tissues. Used in hair treatments.

BEESWAX - (cera alba) used as an emulsifier and moisturiser.

CARMINE - from crushed beetles. Used in lipsticks, blushes and nail polish.

These are just some of the animal products that are used in cosmetics and toiletries. This isn't here to overwhelm you but instead to show the many different animal products that can sneak into the products we buy. The best course of action is to find brands that are vegan and clearly label their products so that you can more easily make a well-informed decision.

WHAT TO WEAR

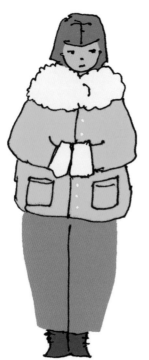

You might have already read the chapter at the beginning of the book that covers reasons not to wear clothing made from animal products. If you haven't then I would highly recommend you do so to educate yourself on the topic.

There are specialised clothing lines that are targeted to vegetarians and vegans and you can easily find them through searching online. However, there is no need to buy all new clothing, as lot of the clothes you probably already own are made from non-animal products like cotton, linen and polyester.

There are plastic and plant alternatives for products such as boots, belts and outerwear, such as recycled plastic, hemp, organic cotton and cork. Plus, more and more companies are creating innovative materials that are vegan and ethical.

These are some animal products that you can look out for when buying new clothing:

- LEATHER
- FUR
- WOOL
- ANGORA

- CASHMERE
- SILK
- DOWN
- FEATHERS

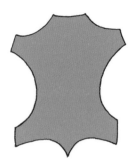

LOOK OUT FOR THIS SYMBOL

Shoes always have a sticker or label telling you what they are made off. The symbol for leather looks like the one above.

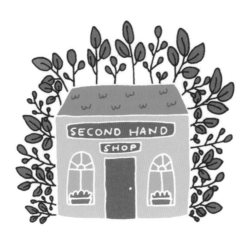

ECO

If you want to opt for the most eco friendly clothing choice buying second-hand is the best, followed by buying ethically-produced clothing.

What about animal items I already own?

A lot of vegans will keep items that they already own and replace them with natural fabrics once they wear out. The environmental impact of completely getting rid of usable clothing and replacing it with new items is far worse than keeping your current items and replacing them with vegan substitutes once they wear out. However, it is completely up to you, as some people no longer feel comfortable wearing animal products after becoming aware of the suffering behind the clothing. If that is the case, make sure that you find a new home for your clothes and don't just throw them in the bin.

CLEANING PRODUCTS

Cleaning products are often tested on animals and they can also be made from animal products. On top of that, a lot of them contain very harsh chemicals that have a negative impact on planet ecology and our health.

Look out for the leaping bunny logo for products that aren't tested on animals, but beware as the leaping bunny doesn't necessarily mean that the product is vegan. Sometimes animal products such as whey sneak into the ingredients. There are other animal products that can sneak in, from beeswax to animal lecithin, which comes from the nervous tissue.

Instead of spending time checking the ingredients, it is easier to go for brands that are vegan, such as the Co-op's own range or Method. If you are unsure whether a brand is vegan, a quick internet search will give you all the info you need.

However, if you are looking to simplify and make your cleaning as ethical as possible, there are DIY options that can reduce the number of harsh chemicals in your home and the amount of plastic you consume, whilst still having a squeaky clean home.

LOW IMPACT DIY
POWERFUL CLEANERS

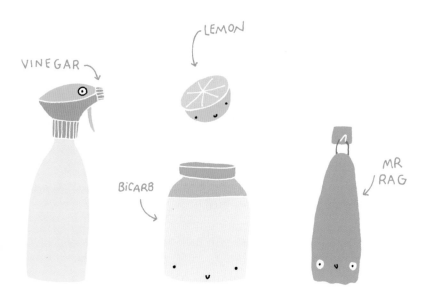

VINEGAR

LEMON

BiCARB

MR RAG

Diluted vinegar, bicarbonate of soda and lemon are powerful everyday cleaners. Castile soap can also be diluted to use as a general surface cleaner. Bicarb can be used to clean tough grease in the oven but can also double up as an air freshener when mixed with essential oils. When cleaning windows, newspaper and a mixture of distilled white vinegar, rubbing alcohol and water works a treat.

VEGAN COMMUNITY

There is a community for everyone and they come in many forms, from online communities to groups that meet in your area.

Community is important for a compassionate and cohesive society.

Going vegan can be a bit overwhelming to begin with, and having a community and/or a vegan friend can make all the difference.

Vegan communities will not only help you find like-minded people, you will also get to know all the local vegan info. So vegan markets, cafés, restaurants, activities, pot-lucks and much more could all be at the tips of your fingers!

If you are not on social media, you can still find events through Meetup.com, or set up your own if there isn't already one in place! Another alternative is volunteering at an animal sanctuary as you are bound to meet fellow vegans and animal lovers.

Here a some of the online communities that you
could become part of:

Vegan Runners
Vegan Pregnancies & Parenting
Vegan Asians
Black Vegans
Vegan Latinos
Zero Waste Vegans
Vegan Activists
Vegan Travellers
Accidentally Vegan Foods
Vegan Bakers
Vegan Kids
Vegan on Budget
Gluten-free Vegans
Vegan Women's Bodybuilding & Fitness
Ask a Vegan Dietitan

In summary, communities are great for
friendship, support and information.

Everything is so much more fun with good
friends!

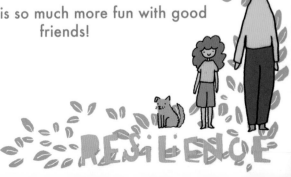

RESILIENCE

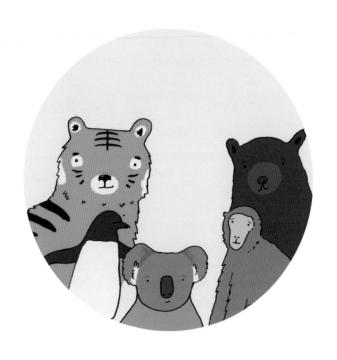

ZOOS &
AQUARIUMS

ANIMAL WELFARE

SPACE - Animals kept in captivity have a tiny percentage of the space that they would have in their natural habitats. Tigers and lions have 18,000 times less space and polar bears have 1 million times less space. Elephants in the wild can walk up to 195km a day.

THEY SUFFER - a lot of animals in zoos display stress behaviour and even depression. A UK study found that 54% of the elephants they studied showed stereotypies (abnormal behaviours due to their needs not being met).

THEY ARE KILLED OR DIE PREMATURELY - A freedom for Animals study found that at least 7,500 animals are deemed as 'surplus' in European zoos. Animals are killed with the excuse that culls are needed. This is on top of the animals who die prematurely due to poor welfare conditions that they face in captivity instead of in the wild.

TRICKS - Animals are forced to perform instead of being allowed to behave normally.

TAKEN - the majority of elephants in European zoos are taken from the wild. Many other species of land, sea and air are made to travel thousands of miles around the world just to be kept in captivity.

Animals in zoos are held in captivity against their will. In the wild, animals will hide away from humans as much as possible as this is their nature. However, zoos are profit-driven and their customers are people who want to actually see the animals, so the animals are made to live in a way where they are forced to display themselves to paying customers.

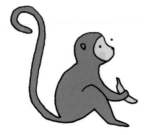

The majority of species in zoos aren't endangered; however, zoos like to advertise to their customers that they are helping with animal conservation as a way to validate keeping animals captive. Furthermore, animals are still being taken from the wild to be put in zoos. The journey that these animals have to endure is unjust. The animals that zoos and aquariums do breed are often of no conservation value due to them being hybrid or unknown subspecies. Zoos offer very little in terms of reintroduction of animals to the wild.

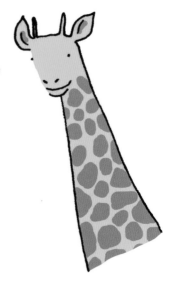

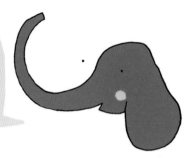

You will learn much more about me from a documentary than you can ever learn from watching me imprisoned, plus you won't be supporting my needless suffering!

Education is another reason that zoos use to legitimise their existence. However animals in zoos do not behave naturally because they are not in their natural habitats. Much more can be learnt from documentaries where you see and learn about the animal in a much more in-depth way. A study in 2010 found that there is no conclusive evidence that shows that zoos and aquariums have an educational impact on visitors. Animal sanctuaries or wildlife habitats are a great alternative for a family day out where you can have the pleasure of seeing an animal lead their natural lives whilst also supporting a good cause.

GLASS CAGES ARE STILL CAGES

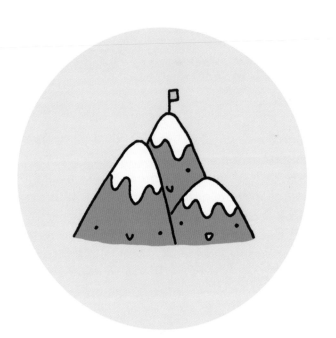

VEGAN
TRAVELLER

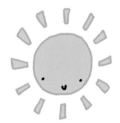
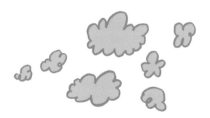

As a new vegan you might be a little scared of travelling as a vegan for the first time, but no need to worry! With a little preparation and know-how, being a vegan traveller will be a piece of (vegan) cake.

Plus, by cutting out the foods that you normally would have consumed, you have opened yourself up to a whole new world of culinary delight. A lot of cultures consume less animal products than we do in the UK and therefore are more adventurous with their food.

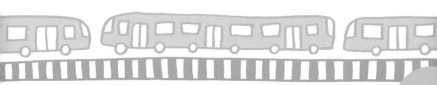

BEFORE TRAVELLING

Follow vegan travel blogs or social media accounts to get inspiration for your next adventure.

If you have a smartphone it is a good idea to download HappyCow, Vanilla Bean, The Vegan Passport and Vaganagogo. The first two find local, vegan-friendly restaurants and supermakerts, and the second two are multilingual vegan phrasebooks. You can use these to see how vegan-friendly a destination is and to familiarise yourself with words such as 'egg' and 'lactose' so as to make it easier when buying food.

Join vegan Facebook groups in your home city and in the city that you are planning on visiting, and either ask for suggestions or look through the page posts for recommendations.

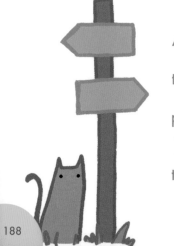

Another trick is to use Instagram or Pinterest: type the name of the city and the word 'vegan' or 'plantbased' restaurant to find places that people have recently gone to. And if you really want to be prepared, email the local tourism association asking about vegan restaurants and shops.

WHILST TRAVELLING

Pack savoury and sweet snacks such as crackers, oat bars, nuts and chocolate for emergencies or to keep the wolf from the door.

Take notes and screenshots of cafés and restaurants you want to visit in case you don't have Wi-Fi whilst out and about.

If you are at a restaurant that doesn't have many vegan options, don't be afraid to let them know of your dietary requirements. A lot of places will be happy to accommodate and adapt something from the menu or create something entirely new.

If you are at a vegan cafe or restaurant and they seem friendly, ask the staff for suggestions for your next meal.

Take a container and cutlery with you in case you want to make lunches or save food for later.

ACCOMMODATION

If you are going all-inclusive contact the provider to make sure that there will be vegan options available.

Airbnbs with kitchens really come in handy for buying local produce and cooking up meals yourself. This makes it easy to visit remote destinations that might not have many restaurants that cater for vegans, and it could save you money.

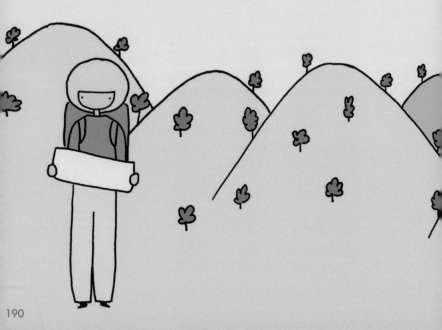

It is possible to find 100% vegan or vegetarian hostels and guesthouses. This could be a great opportunity to cook with like-minded people and share delicious food.

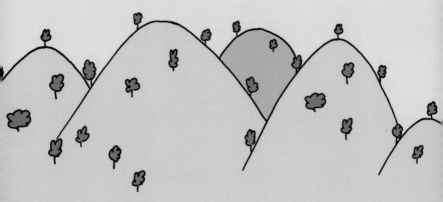

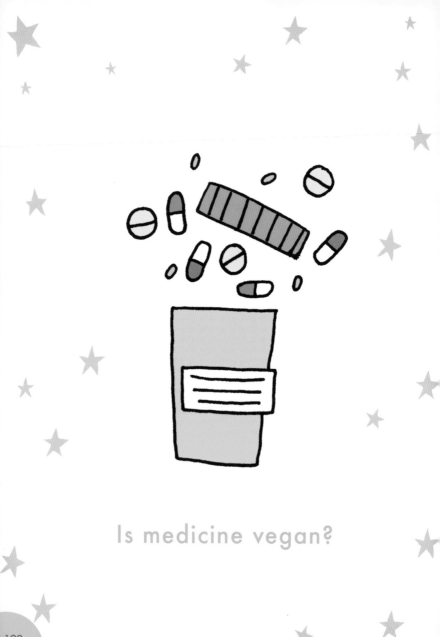

Is medicine vegan?

MEDiCiNE

A lot of medicines are tested on animals and/or contain animal products. However, veganism is a way of living that seeks to avoid exploitation or cruelty to animals as *far as possible*. So if your doctor has prescribed you medicine that contains lactose or comes in gelatine capsules, and if there is no alternative without these animal ingredients, take your medicine and don't feel bad.

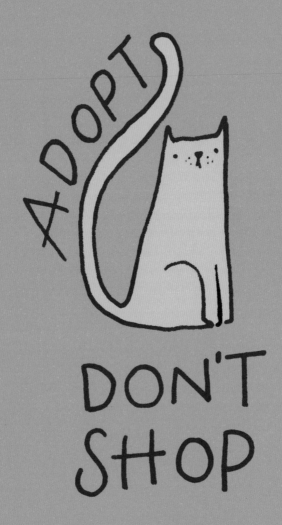

ADOPT
DON'T SHOP

By now it will have become quite clear that veganism it's not just about what what we put in our mouths, although this is a good place to start! Veganism is a way of living more compassionately.

This extends to our pets and where we get them from. There are two main reasons why it is better to adopt than to buy from a breeder. Number one is that every pet that we get from a breeder is a pet that we could have adopted. It's another fluffy animal that is in a shelter wanting a forever home missing out on the opportunity of having a loving family. Number two, by buying from a breeder you are basically paying them to breed more animals into existence when so many are already in need of a home. Not only that, but breeders at the end of the day are making a profit from exploiting animals and that is not right.

LIVING in a NON-VEGAN WORLD

What people tend to find the hardest when going vegan is having to live in a non-vegan world surrounded by omnis (omnivores) who constantly challenge your way of life and ask you hundreds of questions.

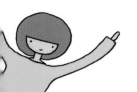
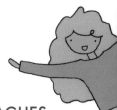

FRIENDS/ACQUAINTANCES/COLLEAGUES

Your relationship with your friends doesn't have to change at all once going vegan. However, most people do experience friends making fun of them a little bit just because there are stereotypes around veganism. In general, veganism can make people quite defensive as they worry that you are judging them for their decisions, so they pre-emptively attack so as to discredit veganism and hence why they aren't vegan themselves. Because if people accept that going vegan is a good thing, then they have to ask themselves the uncomfortable question of why they are not. Coming up with arguments against veganism gets them off the hook. The key here is to stay calm. A lot of times people are looking to get a rise out of you and by staying calm, your answers come across as rational and strong.

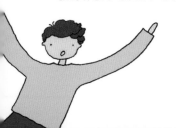
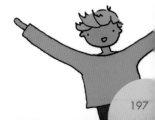

Familiarise yourself with the MYTHS, Q&A and WHY sections of this book, as by having this knowledge you will find it a lot easier to answer any queries people may have. But also remember that you shouldn't be expected to know all the answers, so asking the internet is perfectly ok. Also sometimes you will realise that someone is purposely trying to trip you up and create a nasty environment. It is ok to say that you'd like to stop talking about veganism and that if they are interested they should watch Cowspiracy, or point them towards another source of information that is appropriate to what you were talking about.

Omni friends might feel like they have to accommodate to what they see as limitations, but what they don't realise is that a lot of the time they eat plant-based foods and being vegan is not as complicated as it seems at first. It's as simple as easting Mediterranean dishes or a lentil dhal. Check out the section on eating vegan for more tips.

PARENTS

If you are in the situation where you are living with your parents and they cook for you, your news of going vegan might not be met with a celebration party and seitan burgers. Your parents may worry that you won't get enough protein, calcium, etc. They might also worry that they will have more work on their hands, such as cooking two separate meals. Additionally, they might get defensive that your lifestyle change challenges how they brought you up.

If before going vegan you watched documentaries such as Earthlings, Cowspiracy & Forks over Knives (even better if you watched them with them!), then your family might be more receptive to your change in lifestyle instead of just dismissing it as a "fad" or "phase". Being ready with why you have decided on veganism is important, but it is also important to know how you will go about being vegan in practical terms. Offering to help with the shopping and making meals will go a long way. There is no need for two completely different meals to be made. For example, vegan gravy can be bought for the whole household and the omnis can have animal sausages while you have veggie ones. Spaghetti Bolognese is another example; one can have beef mince and the other can have vegan mince.

All parents are different and all relationships are different, so what might work for someone might not work for the other.

Sometimes no matter how hard you try, family can be not as understanding as we would like them to be. In these cases the best things is to stop using your energy where you are getting no where and instead focus on yourself; focus on why you are vegan and then lead by example, sometimes people just need some time. There are Facebook groups specially for people who live with family who aren't vegan. They can give great advice and tips to living more peacefully with the omnis.

OUT AND ABOUT

Where things might go a bit wrong in our vegan journey is when we are out and about or travelling, and when there are seemingly no vegan options. We are hungry and we falter and get a Mars bar.

First of all, if this happens to you do not be hard on yourself, just view it as a learning curve.

There are some people who manage quite well with not eating for a while. I am not one of these people and, if I don't feed myself regularly, the hunger monster will come out and I will be hangry. This is not nice for me or the people around me. Overtime I have learnt to plan better. For example, if I know that I'm going to be out during lunch time and I plan on getting something out but am not 100% sure that I will be able to, I will pack a couple of snacks or a sandwich, just in case.

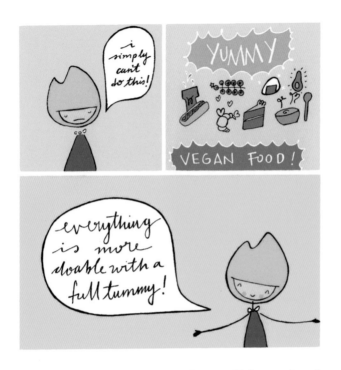

Some snack ideas to keep the wolf from the door:

NUTS - OAT BARS - BISCUITS SUCH AS HOBNOBS, CHOCOLATE CHIP HOBNOBS, OREOS, MOST BOURBONS & TESCO'S DARK CHOCOLATE DIGESTIVES - FRUIT - BAGUETTE WITH HUMMUS - CO-OP DOGHNUTS - CRISPS (CHECK THEY ARE SFV)

Keeping a couple of longlife items in your office cupboard and on your person will save you in a pickle!

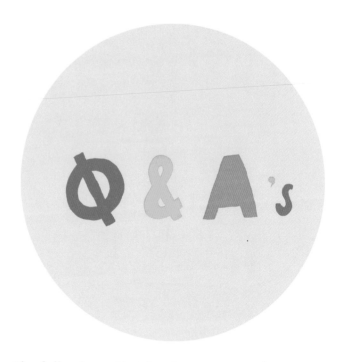

The following will either be questions that vegans are often asked or statements and assumptions that are made about a vegan lifestyle. Being a new vegan can be overwhelming because you are learning a whole new lifestyle. You probably don't have all the answers, but people will challenge you at times – sometimes with questions so ridiculous you couldn't have possibly have predicted them! I have outlined some potential answers that will hopefully help with answering people's curiosity without losing your patience.

Plants feel pain, so what is the point of being vegan anyway?
Plants respond to stimulus but they do not have a nervous system, so they can't feel pain. On the other hand, we know without a doubt that animals do feel physical and emotional pain. And even if we were going to use the 'plants feel pain' argument, then being vegan is still the way of living that causes the least amount of suffering as it takes a lot of plants to feed animals for us to then eat them. We are actually eating fewer plants by not eating animals.

I knew one vegan who was really sick/really horrible...
Vegans come in all forms just like non-vegans. One person doesn't represent all vegans.

I couldn't be vegan because vegans use a lot of soya, and soya production is destroying the rainforest.
Around 90% of soya crops go towards feeding livestock, so by no longer consuming animal products you are also vastly reducing your soya consumption. Furthermore, if you are strongly opposed to soya, you can become one of the many people who are vegan and don't consume any soya.

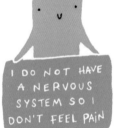

I DO NOT HAVE A NERVOUS SYSTEM SO I DON'T FEEL PAIN

Why do vegans eat things that resemble animal products, such as sausages? Why can't they just eat vegetables?
A lot of vegans enjoyed the taste of animal products, but they stopped eating them because they didn't agree with animals having to die for them. So if they can get products that taste very similar but without the animal suffering, then they will.

So if you were stuck in a desert island with nothing but an animal, would you eat them?

If the animal is there then there must be vegetation that I could eat instead!

However, it is highly unlikely that I will end up on a desert island with nothing to eat but an animal, and this question is only really distracting from our current situation where animals are suffering needlessly for people who think that they are tasty and value their tastebuds over the life of an animal.

Eating animals is my personal choice.
A personal choice is deciding you prefer the colour yellow. It stops being a personal choice when another being comes into the equation. If I punched my friend, saying to them "it's my personal choice" it wouldn't be well received. The same goes with consuming animal products. If you like the colour yellow no one gets hurt and therefore its your personal choice, but if you eat animals products, animals get hurt.

Animals still die in farming your vegetables. Your electronic device was probably produced unethically. and your clothes too.
Sadly this is true. However, there is no perfect way of living that doesn't cause any suffering, but that shouldn't stop us from trying our best. Veganism makes a huge difference in reducing the suffering of sentient beings. Also many more plants are harvested for animal consumption than for direct consumption so numbers of animals dying for vegetables for vegans to eat is still lower. If you can afford to, buying local organic produce is a step further in reducing animal suffering. Buying second-hand is a great way to reduce your consumption of fast fashion, and you can choose to buy from companies that are ethically accredited. However, nit picking and trying to find holes in a person's choice to be vegan doesn't help anyone; we should all try to lift up one another and try to live in a compassionate way.

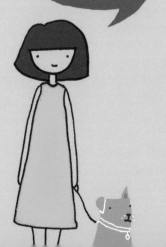
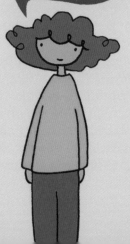

If we don't milk cows it's uncomfortable for them, so milking in necessary.
Dairy cows only exist because we breed them and then impregnate them and separate them from their calf. In nature, they would feed their young and, once the calf was old enough, like humans, the milk production would stop. Cows don't need humans to milk them naturally. However, farmers have selectively bred cows to produce more and more milk, which is painful for them to carry, and the cows are also given hormones. Cows not bred for intensive dairy production do not have this problem as they produce the perfect amount of milk for their babies.

If everyone goes vegan overnight we will be overpopulated with animals!
This is highly unlikely to happen because the world won't go vegan overnight. What has been happening and what will carry on happening is that consumption of animal products is decreasing as more people find out the benefits of a plant-based lifestyle. The animal market works in the same way that other markets work: supply and demand. When demand dips, supply is reduced so as not to produce surplus. This means that less animals will be bred so less animals are born. There's no need to worry that they will overpopulate and take over!

If you have to take B12 supplements, how it is natural?
B12 used to be more present in soil and in vegetables but, due to intensive farming practices and pesticides, there is very little present nowadays. Animals also used to get it from the soil; however, for the same reasons they don't get enough B12, so the farmer supplements their diet too. By taking a B12 supplement you are cutting out the middleman (or should we say, middle cow).

If we didn't farm animals then they wouldn't exist..
There are thousands of species that have gone extinct because of animal farming, so if we are worried about losing animals then we should stop supporting animal agriculture. Also it is preferable for animals to not be bred into existence than for them to be born into world of suffering. Finally, there are a huge number of animal sanctuaries that continuously rescue farm animals and give them a forever home.

Don't we have more important things to worry about such as human rights?
There is no rule that says that you can only pick one cause and to hell with everything else. You can be a vegan and fight for human rights, you can be a vegan and be an environmentalist. You can be a vegan and fight for any cause that you like.

But from an environmental point of view isn't it better to eat locally-produced, grass-fed animal products rather than avocados, fruits and nuts that are from another part of the world, or processed mock meats packed in plastic?
Although it is best when we can to source our plant foods locally and package-free, an Oxford study published in 2018 showed that, from a climate change perspective, even the plant-based diet with the biggest environmental impact was still better than the animal product diet with the lowest environmental impact. If you are concerned about plastic packaging, join a vegan zero waste group online for useful resources.

But I only buy organic animal products, so that's ok. Even organic and free-range farming cause animal suffering. Female cows are impregnated over and over again and have their babies taken away from them so that humans can drink their babies' milk. Male baby cows get slaughtered because they don't produce milk. Male chicks are killed at one day old in the egg industry because they don't lay eggs. Animals undergo various mutilations such as castration and ear-tagging. And finally, even if somehow these animals were well cared-for apart from the things mentioned above, they still get killed prematurely even though they want to live. There there is no way to humanely kill a healthy animal.

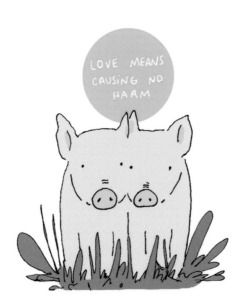

LOVE MEANS CAUSING NO HARM

vegan
ETiQUETTE

Once you've found out all the atrocities about animal agriculture and you've been vegan for a while, it is easy to forget that we were once meat-eating, cow breast milk drinkers. It is also easy to forget that being vegan is easy because you've already taken the hard steps.

We have to remember that we are in a non-vegan society, where big corporations benefit from keeping things how they are, meaning they want to carry on exploiting animals to make money. People have grown up being told that they need to drink that glass of milk for the strength of their bones simply because of a scheme funded by the dairy industry.

All our lives we have been fed the message that it is necessary and normal to eat animals.

So please be kind to your omni friends and family. Lead by example that you can have a full and healthy life as a vegan. If they show an interest, engage with them how you would have liked before you were vegan. Show them some documentaries. Sow seeds and be patient; if people feel like you are pushing it is human nature for them to stand their ground and push back.

Of course, if people are being rude to you, then you don't have to have to take it! Walk away. Ain't nobody got time for that.

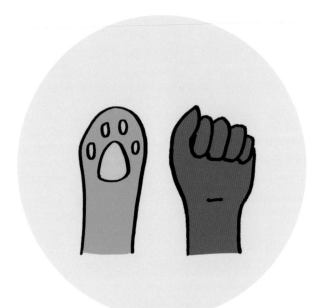

VEGAN
ACTiViSM

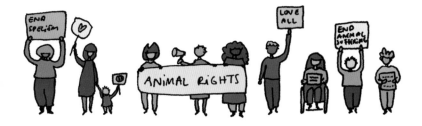

Once we find out the hard truths of the animal industry and the benefits of veganism, it is understandable that we get angry at the injustices that are so insidious in our everyday life. From the dissonance of your loved ones to simply seeing dead animals all around us. Anger in itself is not a bad thing; it's what we do with it that matters. There is no use in getting angry at our relatives and friends, as anger makes people put up walls and shut out what we have to say, however truthful it is. Anger comes from feeling powerless, so instead of directing our anger towards our loved ones let's harness it into something productive and effective like activism.

Not only will you be making a difference, but it is also a chance to meet more vegans and get inspired.

Different types of activism:
Protests/demonstrations - Marches - Free vegan food sample events - Chalktivism - Encouraging businesses to have more vegan options - Joining or creating vegan communities - Donating - Making vegan food for friends and family - Online campaigns - Vigils - Artivism

Vegan activism organisations:
Vegan Outreach - The Save Movement - Voice for the Anonymous - The Earthlings Experience - Viva - Hunt Saboteurs Association - Cube of Truth

Find local activism events near you through the internet, or ask your local vegan group for suggestions. Don't worry if you haven't had any previous experience as it is an opportunity to grow, learn, make new friends and have new experiences.

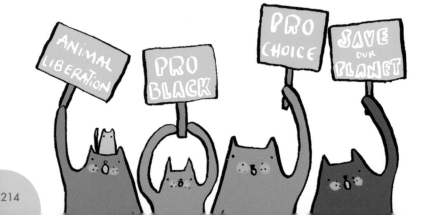

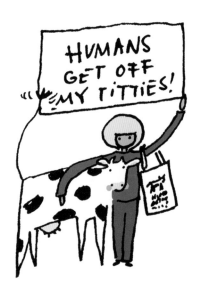

If you are going to events where you are directly talking to people, then I would recommend that you read the Q&A, myths and the first chapter of this book to help you get ready for whatever questions the public might have. I've found that watching YouTube videos of activists in action will make you more familiar and confident with how one-to-one activism works.

Every action, big or small, has the possibility to be a positive impact on the world. Together we can make a big difference!

EXTENDING OUR COMPASSION

I have always had my doubts about what difference one person can make. But after going vegan and seeing the impact of my lifestyle choice in statistics, such as how much less I contribute to greenhouse gases and how many animals a year I would have been responsible for killing had I not gone vegan, I know that my choices make a difference. Additionally, I have many friends who have taken up veganism and many more who are reducing their animal products. I would like to think that, just like how my friend back at uni helped me go vegan, I too have helped other people.

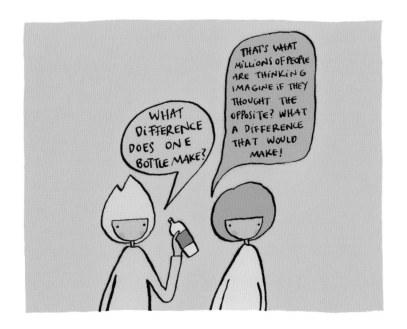

So we definitely know that we can make a difference! Realising this has motivated me to make other changes that I had not had the motivation or knowledge in the past to do. I've quit fast fashion and now buy 90% of my clothes second-hand, because I learnt, from the documentary True Cost, of the horrific working conditions for people abroad and in the UK. I have tried to reduce my plastic consumption by taking steps such as always carrying a water bottle with me and using my own carrier bags. I do this because 100,000 marine mammals and 1 million sea birds die each year because of plastic pollution.

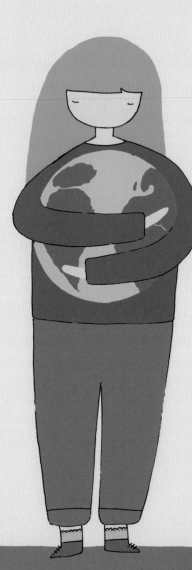

TOGETHER
WE CAN
MAKE A
DIFFERENCE
FOR THE
BETTER.

FOR PEOPLE,
ANIMALS &
THE PLANET.

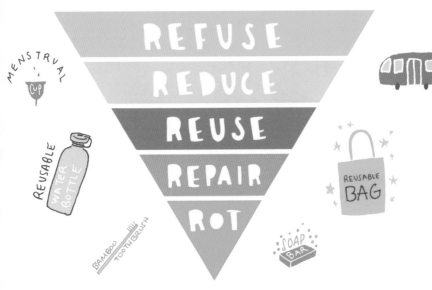

Simply cutting out fast fashion or going full-on zero waste might not be feasible for everyone for different reasons, but simply starting to be aware of these issues and making more conscious decisions which we know can make a difference will go a long way. Some ideas are:

- Reducing fast fashion purchases and opt for second-hand or ethical where possible
- Reducing flights and using trains and buses
- Using a menstrual cup or period underwear instead of disposable sanitary products

RESOURCES

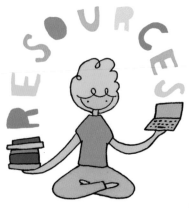

PODCASTS

The Chickpeeps
BHL Fit Club
Brown Vegan
Nutrition Facts
Food for Thought
Our Hen House
Ordinary Vegan Podcast
Vegan Society
The Bearded Vegans

BOOKS

-Eating Animals
-The Sexual Politics
of Meat
-Animal Liberation
-Why We love Dogs, Eat
Pigs, and Wear Cows
-How Not to Die
-Becoming Vegan: The
Complete Reference on
Plant-based Nutrition
-Sistah Vegan

WEBSITES

barnivore.com
nutritionfacts.org
pcrm.org
onegreenplanet.org
plantbasednews.org
viva.org.uk
blackvegansrock.com
happycow.net

APPS

Happy Cow
Finds places to eat near you.
VeganXpress
Helps you find vegan options in chains and fast food restaurants in the USA.
Veganagogo
Helps you find restaurants, order food and explain your dietary requirements in the local language.
Vegan Passport
Created by The Vegan Society to help you travel as a vegan.

Food Monster
1000s of vegan and allergy-friendly recipes.
21-Day Vegan Kickstart
Recipes and tips.
Oh She Glows
Comprehensive archive of delicious recipes.

Is it Vegan? - Animal-Free - Vegan Pocket - Bunny Free - Cruelty-Free
Apps that can tell you wether a product is vegan!
Vegaholic
From the people who made Barnivore, this app allows you to find out whether your alcohol of choice is vegan!

REFERENCES

ANIMALS

www.veganuary.com/why/animals

www.ciwf.org.uk/farm-animals

www.foodispower.org

AHDP. (2017). Baseline report: 2013-2016 Measuring welfare outcomes in pigs.

AHDB. (2018). Fourth Report, GB Cattle Health & Welfare Group.

Brown, C. (2014). Fish intelligence, sentience and ethics. *Animal Cognition*, 18(1), pp.1-17.

Hagen, K. and Broom, D. (2004). Emotional reactions to learning in cattle. *Applied Animal Behaviour Science*, 85(3-4), pp.203-213.

Lymbery, P. (2002). In too deep: the welfare of intensively farmed fish. A compassion in world farming report.

von Keyserlingk, M. et al. (2009). Invited review: The welfare of dairy cattle—Key concepts and the role of science. *Journal of Dairy Science*, 92(9), pp.4101-4111.

Žydelis, R., Small, C. and French, G. (2013). The incidental catch of seabirds in gillnet fisheries: A global review. *Biological Conservation*, 162, pp.76-88.

ZOOS

Clubb, R. and Mason, G. (2002). A review of the welfare of elephants in European zoos. Horsham, UK: RSPCA.

Harris, M. et al. (2008). The welfare, housing and husbandry of elephants in UK zoos. Final report. UK: University of Bristol.

Malamud, R. et al. (2010). Do zoos and aquariums promote attitude change in visitors? A critical evaluation of the american zoo and aquarium study. *Society & Animals*, 18(2), pp.126-138.

ENVIRONMENT

www.cowspiracy.com

Hertwich, E. et al. (2010). Assessing the environmental impacts of consumption and production: priority products and materials. A Report of the Working Group on the Environmental Impacts of Products and Materials to the International Panel for Sustainable Resource Management. UNEP.

IPCC. (2018). Global warming of 1.5°C. An IPCC Special Report on the impacts of global warming of 1.5°C above pre-industrial levels and related global greenhouse gas emission pathways, in the context of strengthening the global response to the threat of climate change, sustainable development, and efforts to eradicate poverty

Poore, J. and Nemecek, T. (2018). Reducing food's environmental impacts through producers and consumers. *Science*, 360(6392), pp.987-992.

Springmann, M. et al. (2016). Analysis and valuation of the health and climate change cobenefits of dietary change. *Proceedings of the National Academy of Sciences*, 113(15), pp.4146-4151.

Steinfeld, H. (2006). Livestock's long shadow. Rome: Food and agriculture organization of the United Nations.

Tilman, D. and Clark, M. (2014). Global diets link environmental sustainability and human health. *Nature*, 515(7528), pp.518-522.

U.S. Environmental Protection Agency. (2004). Risk assessment evaluation for concentrated animal feeding operations.

HEALTH

www.veganhealth.org

Aune, D. et al. (2014). Dairy products, calcium, and prostate cancer risk: a systematic review and meta-analysis of cohort studies. *The American Journal of Clinical Nutrition*, 101(1), pp.87-117.

Dinu, M. et al. (2016). Vegetarian, vegan diets and multiple health outcomes: A systematic review with meta-analysis of observational studies. *Critical Reviews in Food Science and Nutrition*, 57(17), pp.3640-3649.

Fernandez-Cao, J. et al. (2013). Heme iron intake and risk of new-onset diabetes in a Mediterranean population at high risk of cardiovascular disease: an observational cohort analysis. *BMC Public Health*, 13(1).

Hu, J. et al. (2011). Dietary cholesterol intake and cancer. *Annals of Oncology*, 23(2), pp.491-500.

McMacken, M. and Shah, S. (2017). A plant-based diet for the prevention and treatment of type 2 diabetes. *Journal of Geriatric Cardiology*, 14(5), pp. 342–354.

Park, S. et al. (2014). A milk protein, casein, as a proliferation promoting factor in prostate cancer cells. *The World Journal of Men's Health*, 32(2), p.76.

Zeng, S. et al. (2015). Egg consumption is associated with increased risk of ovarian cancer: Evidence from a meta-analysis of observational studies. *Clinical Nutrition*, 34(4), pp.635-641.

Zhu, B. et al. (2015). Dietary legume consumption reduces risk of colorectal cancer: evidence from a meta-analysis of cohort studies. *Scientific Reports*, 5(1).

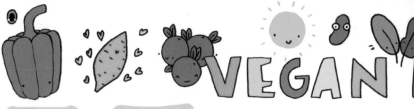

VEGAN

VITAMIN A

Carrots
Sweet Potato
Butternut Squash
Kale & Spinach
Black eyed beans
Turnip Greens
Red Pepper
Mango
Cantaloupe
Grapefruit
Broccoli
Pumpkin

VITAMIN B GROUP

Nutritional Yeast
Whole Grains
Nuts
Leafy Greens
Avocado
Mushrooms
Seeds
Sweet Potato
Wheat Germ
Fortified Foods
Peas
Legumes

VITAMIN B12

Fortified plant-based foods, such as m*lks and cereals, tend to have B12 added to them. Nutritional Yeast has B12 naturally.

Getting enough B12 every day is very important, so taking a B12 supplement is a good idea.

VITAMIN C

Oranges
Peppers
Strawberries
Blackcurrants
Broccoli
Pineapple
Brussels Sprouts
Lemon
Cabbage
Thyme
Cauliflower
Grapefruit

IRON

Lentils
Chard
Molasses
Tofu
Red Kidney Beans
Potatoes
Peas
Chickpeas
Spinach
Oats
Tomatoes
Mushroom

ZINC

Sunflower Seeds
Tofu
Almonds
Hummus
Pumpkin Seeds
Oats
Cashews
Wholewheat Bread
Lentils
Sesame Seeds
Peas
Rice

IODINE

Sea vegetables contain very high levels of iodine, so only a sprinkling of them is needed

Some iodine is present in:

Cranberries
Corn
Potatoes
Bananas
Prunes
Leafy Greens
Lima Beans

MAGNES

Green Leafy
Avocado
Edamam
Cacao Pov
Pumpkin Se
Black Bec
Kidney Be
Soya Bea
Soy Mil
Nuts & Nut E
Wholegrain Bre
Oats
Potatoe
Banana

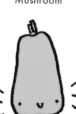
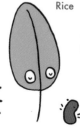
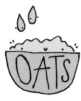
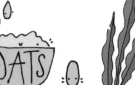